Medical Filing,
2nd edition

Medical Filing,
2nd edition

Terese Claeys, RRA

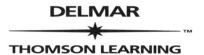

DELMAR

TM

THOMSON LEARNING

Africa • Australia • Canada • Denmark • Japan • Mexico • New Zealand • Philippines
Puerto Rico • Singapore • Spain • United Kingdom • United States

Cover Design: Charles Cummings Advertising/Art, Inc.

Delmar Staff

Publisher: Susan Simpfenderfer
Acquisitions Editor: Marlene Pratt
Project Editor: William Trudell
Marketing Manager: Darryl L. Caron

Art and Design Coordinator: Rich Killar
Production Coordinator: Cathleen Berry
Editorial Assistant: Sarah Holle

COPYRIGHT © 1997
Delmar is a division of Thomson Learning. The Thomson Learning logo is a registered trademark used herein under license.

Printed in the United States of America
12 13 14 15 XXX 06 05 04 03

For more information, contact Delmar Learning, Executive Woods, 5 Maxwell Drive, Clifton Park, NY 12065; or find us on the World Wide Web at http://www.delmar.com

International Division List

Japan:
Thomson Learning
Palaceside Building 5F
1-1-1 Hitotsubashi, Chiyoda-ku
Tokyo 100 0003 Japan
Tel: 813 5218 6544
Fax: 813 5218 6551

Australia/New Zealand:
Nelson/Thomson Learning
102 Dodds Street
South Melbourne, Victoria 3205
Australia
Tel: 61 39 685 4111
Fax: 61 39 685 4199

UK/Europe/Middle East:
Thomson Learning
Berkshire House
168-173 High Holborn
London
WC1V 7AA United Kingdom
Tel: 44 171 497 1422
Fax: 44 171 497 1426

Latin America:
Thomson Learning
Seneca, 53
Colonia Polanco
11560 Mexico D.F. Mexico
Tel: 525-281-2906
Fax: 525-281-2656

Canada:
Nelson/Thomson Learning
1120 Birchmount Road
Scarborough, Ontario
Canada M1K 5G4
Tel: 416-752-9100
Fax: 416-752-8102

Asia:
Thomson Learning
60 Albert Street, #15-01
Albert Complex
Singapore 189969
Tel: 65 336 6411
Fax: 65 336 7411

Library of Congress Catloging-in-Publication Data
Claeys, Terese
  Medical Filing / Terese Claeys — 2nd ed.
    p.   cm.
  Includes bibliographical references and index.
  ISBN: 0-8273-8177-8
  1. Medical records. 2. Files (Records) I. Title
  [DNLM: 1. Forms and Records Control. 2. Medical Records W80
C583m 1996]
R864.C53 1996
651.5'04261—dc20
DNLM/DLC   96-9526
for Library of Congress   CIP

Contents

C

Preface

An organized filing system for medical facilities is necessary for retrieval of medical records. *Medical Filing* is a twelve to fifteen hour unit addressing all types of medical filing. This text-workbook can be used alone or in conjunction with other texts in courses where medical filing is taught. It may be used in community colleges, technical institutions, in-service training, or any office procedures course where medical filing concepts are presented to medical assistants, medical secretaries, dental assistants, medical records technicians, or medical office personnel. The text-workbook will be able to serve as a reference on the job when organizing filing systems.

Topics covered in *Medical Filing* include numeric filing, alphabetic filing, cross-referencing, color coding, records control, and computer-assisted filing. The text-workbook consists of seven short units. Each unit begins with objectives and a short overview to help students focus on the main concepts of the unit. Examples and illustrations appear throughout. Check Your Understanding exercises appear within units to assist students in their understanding of the filing concepts as they are presented. Answers to Check Your Understanding exercises are included at the end of the text-workbook. Each unit ends with Check Your Knowledge exercises. Hands-on application projects are included for alphabetic filing, numeric filing, (consecutive, middle-digit, and terminal-digit), and color coding. These application projects, entitled Apply Your Knowledge, give students real-life experience.

Medical Filing includes the following important features.

■ It is a short, all-inclusive unit on medical filing, making it flexible and, therefore, appropriate for a variety of teaching situations.

■ All types of medical filing are addressed, including computer concepts in the medical office or facility.

■ Filing rules are compatible with Association of Records Managers and Administrators (ARMA) guidelines.

■ Hands-on applications of filing rules provide students with practical experience.

■ All necessary supplies are included in the text-workbook except for a pencil and envelopes for the application project filing cards.

An instructor's manual is available, which includes teaching suggestions and transparency masters for each unit and answers to Check Your Understanding, Check Your Knowledge, and Apply Your Knowledge exercises. It is organized to follow the material in the text-workbook. The instructor's manual also includes a comprehensive final exam and a final application project with answers. The final application project includes a combination of alphabetic and numeric filing methods and cross-referencing.

The revised edition of *Medical Filing* is enhanced by the addition of several new topics. Additional topics include alternate storage methods of health records including the computerized patient record, phonetic filing and automated tracking system. More exercises have been added throughout the text workbook to assist students in understanding the concepts. A Glossary has also been added. The first time key terms are used in the text-workbook they appear in bold letters. All of these terms are included in the Glossary. Need to know terms are in italics in the workbook. The instructor's manual includes additional teaching suggestions along with transparency masters for new concepts addressed.

The author wishes to acknowledge important contributors to the revision of this text-workbook - especially Joanne Becker for her support and encouragement. I would like to extend special thanks to the following reviewers:

- Paula Michal, BSN, Santa Barbara Business College, Santa Barbara, California

- Michele Green, CMA, RRA, ART, Alfred State College, Alfred, New York

- Jerri Adler, CMA, CMT, Lane Community College, Eugene, Oregon

- Estella Gorecki, Northwest Technical Institute, Springdale, Arkansas

- Faye Thompson, Formerly of Cincinnati School of Court Reporting, Cincinnati, Ohio

Terese Claeys

Unit 1

Medical Filing: An Overview

Objectives

After completing this unit, you will be able to:

1. Identify the purpose of medical filing.

2. Identify the five phases of the medical records life cycle and give examples of each phase.

3. Describe the purpose of confidentiality and identify who has control of information being released.

4. Identify and describe two methods of storing medical records.

5. Define cross-referencing.

6. Describe the master patient index.

7. Identify the three most common pieces of storage equipment used for medical filing.

8. Identify and describe three filing supplies used for medical filing.

9. Identify and describe alternative storage methods for patient health records.

An organized filing system for the medical office or medical facility is necessary for retrieval of medical records. A **medical record** is a permanent written document containing pertinent facts about a patient's illnesses and treatments. The medical record contains information identifying the patient and documents the patient's and family's history, physical findings, results of testing, diagnoses, and treatments.

The medical record is beneficial to the patient, health care provider, and public. It benefits the patient by serving as a reference on illnesses and treatments allowing for continuity of care. This provides information to third party payers for financial reimbursement and protects legal interests of the patient in situations such as those involving personal injury and workmen's compensation cases. Health care providers use the information in the medical record to manage patient care. Medical record documentation by health care professionals assists in protecting their legal interests, for example, in malpractice cases. The medical record is beneficial to the public in its contribution to research evaluating treatment and gathering statistical data that may determine current health trends warranting state, federal or world health programs, such as immunization programs.

PURPOSE OF MEDICAL FILING

An efficient filing system is important for the maintenance, retrieval, and security of medical records and health information in order that the medical record is available when needed. For example, for a physician to manage patient care, reference to the medical record for past treatments and history is necessary. The medical record is as much a tool to the health care provider as is a stethoscope. If a medical record is not available, it can lead to duplication of services, such as ordering laboratory tests and x-rays already done. Duplication can be an increased expense to the patient and may be harmful to the patient in some cases. No single filing system is superior; but an understanding of the various types will assist in adopting a filing system that best fits the needs of the health facility.

THE MEDICAL RECORDS LIFE CYCLE

Medical records have a life cycle that begins with the creation of the medical record and ends with its disposition. Figure 1.1 illustrates the life cycle of medical records.

Figure 1.1
Medical Records
Life Cycle

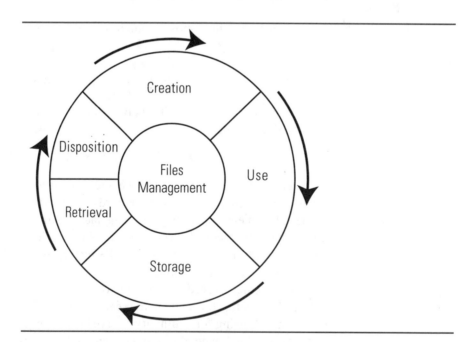

Creation of Medical Records

This is the beginning of the cycle. It starts when information is collected from the patient. This information includes identification data as well as medical information such as past illnesses, allergies, and family history.

Use of Medical Records

Medical records are used for a variety of functions, such as planning and evaluating patient care, obtaining financial reimbursement from insurance companies, and processing legal claims, such as lawsuits.

Storage of Medical Records

The systematic placement of records in a designated area is records storage. It is important that records be stored in a secure area free from dust, fire, and water damage so that they will be available for future use.

Retrieval of Medical Records

The locating of a medical record is called retrieval. A good storage and records control system is necessary for quick retrieval of medical records.

Disposition of Medical Records

Disposition is the destruction of medical records following the expiration of the retention period. The American Medical Association and the American Health Information Management Association recommend that medical records be kept ten years after the patient is no longer seen at the health care facility if there is no state statute that specifies otherwise. If the patient is a minor, medical records should be kept three years after the patient reaches majority. Medical records must be disposed of by burning or shredding to protect the security of their contents.

CONFIDENTIALITY

Medical records are considered legal documents, and maintaining confidentiality of health information is the responsibility of all who work with the medical records. Patients have the right to expect their medical records and the information in them to be protected from unauthorized disclosure. The patient owns the information in the medical record, but the health care facility owns the medical record. No information can be released without proper authorization from the patient or patient's guardian. Unauthorized disclosure could result in harm to the patient or legal action being brought against the health care worker and facility.

Confidentiality also includes not revealing names of individuals treated in the health facility or discussing patients where others may hear, such as at the front desk in an office or in the cafeteria. Patients and their cases should never be discussed outside the medical facility. For consistency, every medical facility should have policies and procedures regarding release of information.

As of this writing, there is no federal law which governs the patient's access to medical records in all situations. However, the Medical Record Confidentiality Act of 1995 (S1360) is pending in Congress. This legislation is designed to protect patient privacy assuring Americans that their sensitive records are protected. It provides clear federal rules which govern access to medical records as to when and to whom information may be disclosed and a means through which patients may review their medical records. It gives the patient the right to limit disclosure of their medical records for purposes other than treatment and billing. If enacted into law this legislation would provide the healthcare system with a federal standard for handling identifiable health information. The Privacy Act of 1974 protects the privacy of individuals identified in information systems maintained by federal agencies, and gives individuals access to records in these systems. The act includes hospital records of federal government hospitals only. About one half of the states have statutes which guarantee patient access to their health information. When patients review their medical records they become more knowledgeable about their condition. This knowledge will allow them to play an active role and make better informed decisions about their medical care. Their illness may become more realistic and less feared. A suggested procedure when a patient requests access to the medical record is to notify the attending physician. If the attending physician believes patient access to the medical record may be detrimental to the physical and/or mental health of the patient, the information should be communicated to the patient in a form which is most appropriate for the patient. If a patient is reviewing a medical record, a health care professional should review the medical record with the patient to assist in interpreting information and to answer questions. To ensure confidentiality and appropriate patient access to medical records, it is very important to include patient access to health information in release of information policy and procedures.

METHODS OF STORING MEDICAL RECORDS

In order to store records in the most efficient way possible, some type of filing or storing method must be used. The two methods used when storing medical records are the alphabetic storage method and the numeric storage method.

Alphabetic Storage

In **alphabetic filing**, medical records are arranged according to the letters of the alphabet. The dictionary is an example of alphabetical arrangement. Medical records are filed by the first letter of the patient's last name.

No one universal set of rules for alphabetic filing is followed by every business or health facility. The Association of Records Managers and Administrators, Inc., (ARMA) has published *Alphabetic Filing Rules,* containing rules for storing records alphabetically. ARMA is an organization designed to help professionals in records management perform their jobs better and more easily. With the rules recommended by ARMA, businesses have a place to start in setting up an efficient alphabetic storage system. The rules used in this text-workbook are in compliance with ARMA standards.

Alphabetic storage is the most common method. Most medical records systems with fewer than 5,000 records will use the alphabetic storage method.

However, large medical records systems are more simply maintained using a numeric storage system.

Numeric Storage

As the name implies, the **numeric filing** of medical records involves assigning a number to each record and filing it according to one of the various numeric sequences. Two major reasons for using a numeric storage method are the infinite set of numbers available and the ease with which people recognize and use numbers. Another very important advantage, particularly for medical records, is that numeric storage maintains confidentiality as it does not reveal the identity of a patient as easily as the patient name does.

CROSS-REFERENCING

Cross-referencing is preparing an aid that indicates another way a medical record may be filed. In alphabetic filing, a medical record may be requested by a name other than the one indexed. For example, a recently married woman should have her record cross-referenced to her maiden name. Foreign names or names that may be spelled in different ways may also be cross-referenced. In numeric filing, an index with patient names and their medical record numbers must be kept as a cross-reference in order to locate the medical record in the file.

MASTER PATIENT INDEX

The **master patient index** (MPI) is a manual card file or computerized system that contains information on all patients treated by a health facility. The MPI is arranged alphabetically. Minimum data included in a master patient index are patient name, birth date, sex, address, dates of treatment, physician name and medical record numbers. The MPI may serve as a reference for information and for locating the patient's medical record. See Figure 1.2 for a sample format of an MPI card.

The amount of information included in the MPI will depend on the needs of the medical facility. When the patient index is used primarily for locating the patient record, minimum data will be necessary. In a medical facility where the numeric storage method is used, the master patient index is the key to locating the medical record. When retrieving a medical record, the patient name is first looked up in the MPI, the medical record number is identified, and the medical record is then located in the storage area. MPI used in this way is considered a form of cross-referencing.

When the MPI serves as the core of a computerized patient account and clinical data system, more data will be necessary, such as insurance information and diagnoses and procedures for each date of treatment. Keep in mind that entering and storing data is expensive so only information necessary to meet the needs of the facility should be entered.

Figure 1.2
Card from a Master
Patient Index

FAMILY NAME	FIRST NAME	MIDDLE NAME	SEX	AGE	MEDICAL RECORD NUMBER		
Gray	Jerome	Alan	M	89	12-46-50		

ADDRESS			BIRTH DATE	MONTH	DAY	YEAR
112 Western Ave, Gary, IA 52242				06	01	1906

TREATMENT DATE	PHYSICIAN	TREATMENT DATE	PHYSICIAN

FILING EQUIPMENT

The most common types of equipment used for storage are vertical file cabinets, lateral file cabinets, and shelf files.

Vertical File Cabinets

Vertical file cabinets are the conventional one- to five-drawer file cabinets. The popular four-drawer vertical file cabinet is shown in Figure 1.3. In order to open a file drawer all the way, three-foot aisles are required. The advantage of drawer files is that medical records will be dirt- and dust-free. Cabinets can also be locked, adding to security.

Figure 1.3
Vertical File Cabinet

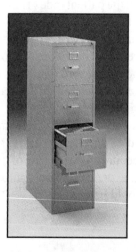

Lateral File Cabinets

Cabinets that have drawers that open from the long side, resembling a chest of drawers, are called lateral file cabinets. They are well-suited to narrow spaces and are available in a variety of sizes. Lateral file cabinets take less space than the conventional file cabinets, are also dirt- and dust-free, and can be locked. A lateral file cabinet is shown in Figure 1.4.

Figure 1.4
Lateral File Cabinet

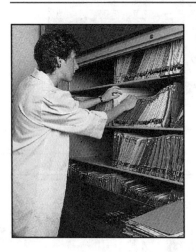

Shelf Files

Shelf files are arranged horizontally. They may be open, have roll-back or roll-down fronts, may be movable on tracks, or be automated. All shelf files are space savers as they hold more records in a given space and require aisle space of 30 to 36 inches. Movable file units save space and usually are considered when storage area is limited as only one fixed aisle is necessary. Access to other aisles is accomplished by manually, mechanically or electrically moving the files on the track to open an aisle where needed. Operating efficiency is increased as the file area is more compact and personnel do not need to walk as far. One drawback is that if the files are highly active, two people cannot work in different areas at the same time. A movable file is shown in Figure 1.5. For easy access, requested records can be retrieved from automated shelf files with a push of the button. Automated files reduce clerical time and energy but access may be inadequate in highly active files. Figure 1.6 shows an automated file. While the automated files are time savers, the movable files save space. The roll-down fronts on the movable files keep the files dust- and dirt-free and can be locked. They are also more expensive than the open-shelf files.

The open-shelf file shown in Figure 1.7 is the most popular method of storing medical records due to efficiency and cost. However, there is a loss of confidentiality with this storage option. Supervising or locking the storage area will increase security.

Figure 1.5
Shelf Files

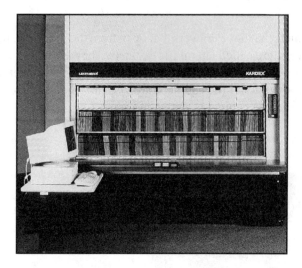

Figure 1.6
Automated File

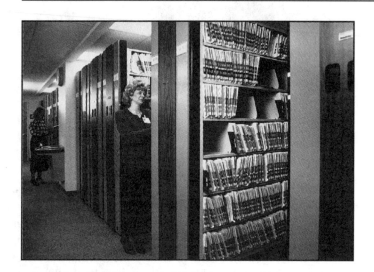

Figure 1.7
Shelf Files

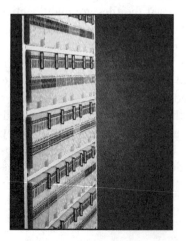

FILING SUPPLIES

Medical records should have protective covers to prevent tearing and loss of reports. Due to easy retrieval, file folders are the most popular covers used.

File Folders

File folders are usually made of heavy material such as manila, plastic, or pressboard and are creased approximately in half with the back higher than the front. They are available with a straight edge or with tabs in various positions. A **tab** is a portion of the folder that extends beyond the regular height or width of the folder. If a tab extends across the complete width or height of a folder, it is said to be a *straight cut* or *full cut*. *Third-cut* tabs extend only one-third of the width of the folder.

Position refers to the location of the tab. *First position* means the tab is at the left; *second position* means the tab is second from the left; and so on. When using file drawers for storage, the tabs will be across the top with either a straight or third cut. When using shelf files, the tab will be along the side of the folder with a straight cut. Study the cuts and tab positions of the folders in Figure 1.8.

Figure 1. 8
Folder Cuts and Tab Positions

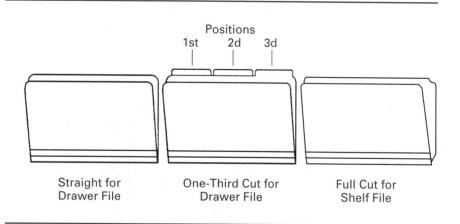

Positions
1st   2d   3d

| Straight for Drawer File | One-Third Cut for Drawer File | Full Cut for Shelf File |

File folders may be purchased with preprinted numbers or letters, which may also be color coded. Fasteners on the inside of the folders to hold the reports in place are another option.

File Guides

File guides should be placed throughout the files for efficient filing and retrieval of medical records. **File guides** are dividers that guide the way to the location of the record being retrieved. Figure 1.9 shows alphabetic file guides. The frequency of the guides depends on the thickness of the individual files. The thicker the folders, the more frequently guides should be placed for ease in locating medical records. Guides should project beyond the record for quick location of records.

Figure 1.9
Alphabetic File Guides

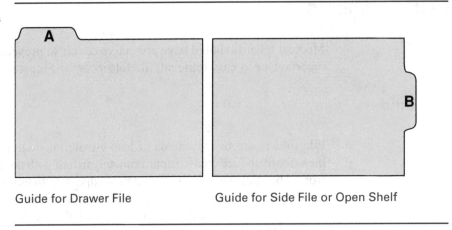

Guide for Drawer File   Guide for Side File or Open Shelf

OUT Guides

To keep track of medical records that are removed from the files, an OUT guide is often used. An **OUT guide** is a card, folder, or sheet of paper temporarily inserted in the file to replace a medical record that has been removed. Use of OUT guides provides a means for record control. The OUT guide indicates the removal date and the record's current location. OUT guides are shown in Figure 1.10.

Figure 1.10
OUT Guides

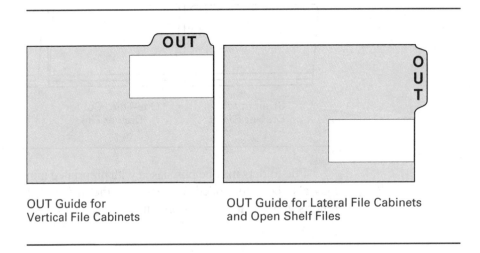

OUT Guide for   OUT Guide for Lateral File Cabinets
Vertical File Cabinets   and Open Shelf Files

When the medical record is being returned to the file, the OUT guide will assist in quickly locating the exact place for the record to be filed. The OUT guide is removed once the medical record is returned to the file. Periodically the OUT guides are checked for medical records that have been removed from the file for a long period of time, usually more than two weeks. These records are then tracked and returned to the file.

ALTERNATE STORAGE METHODS

As storage space decreases and advances in technology continues other storage methods will include microfilming, optical disk storage and computerized patient record.

Microfilming

Microfilming is a photographic process that reduces a document to a very small size. Microfilmed records require very little space, can easily be reproduced, and is a viable option for preservation of health records.

Several storage and retrieval systems are available to access the desired image. They include:

• *roll film* which contains many health records on each roll. It is the least expensive method, cannot be easily updated, is suitable for serially numbered records, and requires manual location of the required health record which is time consuming.

• *cartridges and cassettes* which are similar to roll film. They have the same advantages of roll film without the inconvenience of manual film handling, offer more flexibility but are more expensive.

• *microfilm jackets* which contain transparent material joined horizontally by lines of adhesive which form channels. Microfilmed roll film may be slid into the channels. An advantage of microfilmed jackets is that a unitized patient record may be maintained because it can be updated by inserting new images into the channel.

• *microfiche* which is a sheet of film containing multiple microimages. An advantage is that patient information appears on one sheet rather then a roll. A disadvantage is that new images cannot be added.

• *computer output microfilm* (COM) which takes information stored in a computer on magnetic tape, translates it into readable form, and displays it on a computer display screen. A microfilm camera photographs the displayed information, reducing it to microrecord size and a processor develops the film. The process was developed due to the large quantities of paper that computers generate.

• *computer assisted retrieval* (CASR) is an automated document storage and retrieval system which provides rapid reference to randomly filmed records using computerized indexing and cross-referencing.

Optical Disk Storage

Optical disk storage uses a laser to etch data onto a permanent surface such as prepared glass and can store a vast amount of paper information on a single disk. The system uses a stand alone personal computer, local area network, or large central system. It also includes a scanner to read the documents, high resolution monitors, a "jukebox" that serves to move, without human intervention, optical disks on-line, and a printer or faxing capabilities for output. A disadvantage is the high cost for such a system.

Computerized Patient Record

The health record of the future will be computerized. A **computerized patient record (CPR)** will enhance access and facilitate communication among health care providers at various locations and distances. While there are many benefits, the following problem issues need to be addressed:

- patient privacy and record access
- record ownership
- accreditation and licensure laws that may pose barriers such as requiring entries and signatures to be in ink
- legal risks specific to CPR systems such as unauthorized access to record systems

Computerization of health records will not occur overnight but health care facilities and providers are continually working toward moving from paper records to computerized records.

Student Name

Check Your Knowledge

Directions:
For each of the following situations identify the phase of the medical records life cycle represented and write the term in the space provided.

1.   In the Monday morning mail at Cedar Clinic, a request from Hansen Insurance Company is received for information on Eva Burgos, a former patient. It appears Eva has applied for life insurance. You note proper authorization is included for disclosure of information.

    _____

2.   At the end of each day at Cedar Clinic, the file clerk is responsible for returning medical records to the file.

    _____

3.   New patients at Cedar Clinic are required to complete an information sheet prior to being seen by the physician.

    _____

4.   Each morning prior to patients' visits at Riverside Clinic, the file clerk gathers patient records for the day's appointments.

    _____

5.   The file clerk pulls medical records of patients not seen at Riverside Clinic in more than ten years because they are no longer needed.

    _____

Directions:
In the space provided, fill in the term that fits the definition, description, or question.

6.   Storage equipment for medical records that looks like a chest of drawers and is good for narrow spaces.

    _____

7.   Key to locating the medical record in numeric storage.

    _____

8.   Dividers that assist in the location of medical records.

    _____

This exercise continues on the following page.

9.   Replaces medical records removed from the file.

_____

10.   Who owns the information in the medical record?

_____

11.   A photographic process that reduces a document to a very small size.

_____

12.   A storage and retrieval system which can utilize an unit patient record.

_____

13.   A storage system which uses a laser to etch data onto a permanent surface.

_____

14.   The storage system of future patient records.

_____

Unit 2

Alphabetic Filing

Objectives

After completing this unit, you will be able to:

1. Explain the necessity for indexing rules in alphabetic storage of names and the importance of following these rules consistently.

2. Index and arrange names in indexing order of units.

3. Index and arrange names with punctuation and possessives.

4. Index and arrange names with abbreviations, nicknames, and shortened names.

5. Index and arrange names with prefixes, foreign articles and particles.

6. Index and arrange names with titles and suffixes.

7. Index and arrange names that are identical.

8. Index names for a phonetic filing system.

The most common method of storage is alphabetic. This is the easiest filing system and most commonly used system for organizing medical records in a small facility. When medical records are filed alphabetically, the patient's name is used. File guides for each letter of the alphabet are used as well as guides for some subdivisions for quick location of medical records.

As with any storage system, the alphabetic storage method has advantages and disadvantages. An advantage is that this system is the easiest to learn. Because the system is easy to learn, new personnel in the office can be trained quickly. A disadvantage to filing alphabetically is that names can be misspelled easily. If a name is misspelled, it will be misfiled. Also, when the medical practice expands, each alphabetic section will also expand. This involves shifting medical records in the system to redistribute the space. Another disadvantage is that alphabetic filing makes medical records easily accessible to unauthorized personnel.

ALPHABETIC FILING RULES

To retrieve information efficiently, a set of rules must be followed. The rules in this unit are written to agree with the Association of Records Managers and Administrators, Inc., (ARMA) Simplified Filing Standard Rules and Specific

Filing Guidelines. Variations exist in the procedures for storing records alphabetically. Therefore, the procedures to be used in any office must be determined, recorded, approved, and followed with no deviation. The real test of an efficient storage system is being able to find records once they have been stored.

INDEXING

Indexing means selecting the filing segment under which a record will be filed. The filing segment is the name by which the record is stored and requested. Each filing segment, or name, is broken into units. The key unit is the first unit of the filing segment and the one by which the record is stored. Units 2, 3, 4, and so on, are the subsequent units considered when determining placement of a record in the file.

INDEXING RULES

The rules for alphabetic storage are presented here with examples to help you understand how to apply the rules. Study each rule and the examples carefully; above all, be sure you understand the rule. In determining alphabetic order, compare the units in the filing segment for differences. If the key units of records are alike, move to the second units, the third units, and following units until a difference is found.

Rule 1: Personal Names

Names are indexed in the following order: (1) the last name (surname) is the key unit, (2) the first name (given name or first initial) is the second unit, and (3) the middle name or initial is the third unit. If determining the surname is difficult, consider the last name as the surname. Initials are considered separate indexing units. When a unit consists of just an initial (a single letter), it precedes a unit that consists of a complete name beginning with the same letter. Remember, nothing goes before something. Punctuation is omitted.

Examples: Rule 1

Table 2.1

	Name	Key Unit	Unit 2	Unit 3
1	S. Komuro	KOMURO	S	
2	S. K. Komuro	KOMURO	S	K
3	Sumio Komuro	KOMURO	SUMIO	
4	Sumio T. Komuro	KOMURO	SUMIO	T
5	Sumio U. Komuro	KOMURO	SUMIO	U
6	Sumio Ureko Komuro	KOMURO	SUMIO	UREKO

Check Your Understanding

Check Your Understanding of Rule 1

Directions:
Rewrite the seven personal names below in indexing order according to units. Then alphabetize the names by numbering them from 1-7 on the lines provided.

	Name	Key Unit	Unit 2	Unit 3
____	1. John Meier	_____	_____	_____
____	2. John Robert Meir	_____	_____	_____
____	3. J. Robert Meirs	_____	_____	_____
____	4. J. R. Meir	_____	_____	_____
____	5. Julia Meir	_____	_____	_____
____	6. Julia A. Miers	_____	_____	_____
____	7. Joan K. Meiers	_____	_____	_____

See page 73 for answers.

Rule 2:   Punctuation and Possessives

All punctuation is disregarded when indexing personal names. Commas, periods, hyphens, apostrophes, and dashes are disregarded; and names are indexed as written.

Examples: Rule 2

Table 2.2

	Name	Key Unit	Unit 2	Unit 3
1	Ai-lien Chan	CHAN	AILIEN	
2	Chi-luan Chan	CHAN	CHILUAN	
3	Sylvia Clay-Moore	CLAYMOORE	SYLVIA	
4	J.F. Cruz	CRUZ	J	F
5	Eva M. Cruz-Rivera	CRUZRIVERA	EVA	M
6	Jean Marie D'Andre	DANDRE	JEAN	MARIE
7	Henry F. L'Hendryx	LHENDRYX	HENRY	F

Rule 3:   Abbreviations, Nicknames, and Shortened Names

Abbreviations of personal names (such as, Wm., Jos., Thos.), nicknames (such as, Bud, Guy), and shortened names (such as, Liz, Bill) are indexed as they are written.

Examples: Rule 3

Table 2.3

	Name	Key Unit	Unit 2	Unit 3
1	Mary Johnson	JOHNSON	MARY	
2	Oscar Johnston	JOHNSTON	OSCAR	
3	Will K. Sale	SALE	WILL	K
4	Wm. R. Sale	SALE	WM	R
5	Thos. Sanchez	SANCHEZ	THOS	
6	Tom Sanchez	SANCHEZ	TOM	
7	Jos. Silvas	SILVAS	JOS	
8	Joseph R. Silvas	SILVAS	JOSEPH	R

Rule 4:   Prefixes, Foreign Articles, and Particles

A foreign article or particle in a person's name is combined with the part of the name following it to form a single indexing unit. The indexing order is not affected by a space between a prefix and the rest of the name, and the space is disregarded when indexing. Examples of articles and particles are a la, D', Da, De, Del, De la, Della, Den, Des, Di, Dos, Du, El, Fitz, Il, L', La, Las, Le, Les, Lo, Los, MI, Mac, Mc, O', Per, Saint, San, Santa, Santo, St., Ste., Te, Ten, Ter, Van, Vande, Van der, Von, Von der.

Examples: Rule 4

Table 2.4

	Name	Key Unit	Unit 2	Unit 3
1	DeLore de la Mont	DELAMONT	DELORE	
2	Claude De Monet	DEMONET	CLAUDE	
3	Joel Mac Lean	MACLEAN	JOEL	
4	Joel R. Mc Lean	MCLEAN	JOEL	R
5	John L. Santa Cruz	SANTACRUZ	JOHN	L
6	Teresa Ann St. Clair	STCLAIR	TERESA	ANN
7	Norma J. Van Waus	VANWAUS	NORMA	J
8	Kurt K. Von der Haar	VONDERHAAR	KURT	K

Check Your Understanding

Check Your Understanding of Rules 2, 3, and 4

Directions:
Rewrite the seven names below in indexing order. Alphabetize the list by placing a number from 1-7 in the space provided.

		Name	Key Unit	Unit 2	Unit 3
____	1.	Magdalena Lynch-Weber	_____	_____	_____
____	2.	Carlos D'Cenzo	_____	_____	_____
____	3.	I-chen Liu	_____	_____	_____
____	4.	Jos. Thomas De Andre	_____	_____	_____
____	5.	Will M. St. Vincent	_____	_____	_____
____	6.	Joe Thos D' Amico	_____	_____	_____
____	7.	Carmen Lloyd-Wang	_____	_____	_____

See page 73 for answers.

Rule 5:   Titles and Suffixes

A title before a name (such as, Dr., Miss, Mr., Mrs., Ms., Prof.), a seniority suffix (such as, II, III, Jr., Sr.), or a professional suffix (such as, CRM, DDS, MD, PhD) after a name is the last indexing unit. Numeric suffixes (such as, II, III) are filed before alphabetic suffixes (such as, Jr., PhD, Sr.). If a name contains both a title and a suffix, the title is the last unit. Royal and religious titles followed by either a given name or a surname only (such as, Father Leo) are indexed and filed as written. When royal or religious titles are followed by both a given name and a surname the title is indexed last (such as Sister Monica Riley).

Examples: Rule 5

Table 2.5

	Name	Key Unit	Unit 2	Unit 3	Unit 4
1	Bother Faherty	BROTHER	FAHERTY		
2	J. R. Light, II	LIGHT	J	R	II
3	J. R. Light, III	LIGHT	J	R	III
4	J. R. Light, Jr.	LIGHT	J	R	JR
5	J. R. Light, Sr.	LIGHT	J	R	SR
6	Senora Monica Lopez	LOPEZ	MONICA	SENORA	
7	Queen Margaret	QUEEN	MARGARET		
8	Sister Monica Riley	RILEY	MONICA	SISTER	
9	Jan R. Rivera, CMA	RIVERA	JAN	R	CMA
10	Sen. Jan R. Rivera	RIVERA	JAN	R	SEN

Check Your Understanding

Check Your Understanding of Rule 5

Directions:
Rewrite the seven names below in indexing order. Alphabetize the list by placing a number from 1-7 in the space provided.

	Name	Key Unit	Unit 2	Unit 3	Unit 4
____	1. Dr. Victor S. Perez	____	____	____	____
____	2. Father Tom K. Goedken	____	____	____	____
____	3. Sister Loretta	____	____	____	____
____	4. Jose F. Hernandez, Senior	____	____	____	____
____	5. Jose F. Hernandez, II	____	____	____	____
____	6. Prof. Clark Tirado, Ph.D.	____	____	____	____
____	7. King Harald V	____	____	____	____

See page 73 for answers.

Rule 6:   Identical Names of Persons

If all units, including titles, in the names of two or more persons are identical, filing order is determined by addresses. Cities are considered first, followed by states or provinces (considered by their two letter abbreviated form), street names, and then house numbers or building numbers. Zip codes are not considered in indexing.

Numbers spelled out (such as, seven) are filed alphabetically. Numbers written in digit form are filed before alphabetic letters or words (7 comes before one). Numbers written in digits are filed in ascending (lowest to highest) order. Arabic numerals are filed before Roman numerals (2, 3, II, III).

In some medical facilities, dates of admission or birth dates may be used rather than addresses when names are identical. The latest admission date or birth date is usually sequenced first. The key is consistency.

Examples: Rule 6 *Birth Dates Used to Determine Filing Order*

Table 2.6

	Name	Key Unit	Unit 2	Unit 3	Unit 4	Unit 5
1	Joel Carson Birth Date: August 20, 1989	CARSON	JOEL	1989	AUGUST	20
2	Joel Carson Birth Date: March 20, 1989	CARSON	JOEL	1989	MARCH	20
3	Joel Carson Birth Date: April 11, 1954	CARSON	JOEL	1954	APRIL	11
4	Joel Carson Birth Date: April 30, 1939	CARSON	JOEL	1939	APRIL	30

Table 2.7

Examples: Rule 7 *Addresses Used to Determine Filing Order*

	Name	Key Unit	Unit 2	Unit 3	Unit 4	Unit 5	Unit 6	Unit 7	Unit 8
1	Nancy Lane 1234 5th St. Marion, NV	LANE	NANCY	MARION	NV	5	ST	1234	
2	Nancy Lane 2700 5th St. Marion, WY	LANE	NANCY	MARION	WY	5	ST	2700	
3	Nancy Lane 198 Main ST. Marion, WY	LANE	NANCY	MARION	WY	MAIN	ST	198	
4	Nancy Lane 190 W. Main St. Marion, WY	LANE	NANCY	MARION	WY	W	MAIN	ST	190

Check Your Understanding

Check Your Understanding of Rule 6

Directions:
Alphabetize the names by numbering them from 1-7 on the line next to the name.

_____ 1.   Ms. Amanda K. Fransen, 1120 E. Main, Lansing, IA

_____ 2.   Paul John Lansing, St. Paul, MN

_____ 3.   Amanda K. Fransen, 112 W. Main, Lansing, IA

_____ 4.   Paul John Lansing, St. Paul, MI

_____ 5.   Miss Anna Maria Franks

_____ 6.   Mr. D. M. LaBrie, Ely, NV

_____ 7.   Delora LaBrie, 18 Pine Tree Ave., Ely, MN

See page 73 for answers.

PHONETIC FILING

Phonetic filing may be used by health facilities where there is a greater diversity of last names in the community. **Phonetic filing** is a system in which all surnames that sound alike but are spelled differently are filed together. Names are not indexed by exact spelling but name variations are brought together by use of a code number which represents key letters. The first letter of the last name is retained for the primary order of filing and then the next three consonants or key letters are translated into a three digit code. Similar sounding consonants use the same code number. Code assignment is as follows:

Consonants	Code Assignment
b, f, p, v	1
c, g, j, k, q, s, x, z	2
d, t	3
l	4
m, n	5
r	6

In the phonetic system the vowels *a, e, i, o, u,* and *y* are separators. When consonants having the same number assignment are separated by a vowels or *y* they are coded individually. The letters *w* and *h* are not separators and are not coded. There are five rules to follow in phonetic filing:

1. When two or more consonants with the same code assignment occur together, treat them as one letter.
2. If a name contains less than three consonants, add zeros to arrive at the code number.
3. If two consonants having the same code number assignment appear together and are separated by a vowel or *y*, the consonants are coded separately.
4. It two consonants with the same code assignment are separated by an *h* or *w*, code one consonant.
5. After coding of the surname, arrangement between the key letter guides should be alphabetical according to the given name.

An advantage of phonetic filing is that the user does not have to think of the various ways a name may be spelled when searching for a record. Sponsors of this system claim that this method detects duplication in the files and discloses 90 percent of all transposition of letters. A disadvantage is the time involved in training.

Many computerized systems offer the phonetic capability of searching the Master Patient Index. When a patient's name is typed into the computer system all possible names will be displayed along with other identifiable information. If the name Anderson is typed, other possible ways of spelling the name will appear such as Andersen, Andreson, etc. The user will not need to retype the various ways a name is spelled.

Examples of Names in a Phonetic Filing System

Name	Primary File Order	Secondary File Order
Atwater Brewster	A360	Brewster
Barkema, Lin A.	B625	Lin A
Bielejeski, Ramon	B422	Ramon
Hommerding, Tosha K.	H563	Tosha
Puskin, Charles	P250	Charles
Schmidt, Adolph	S530	Adolph

Check Your Understanding

Check Your Understanding of Rule 6

Directions:

Translate the following alphabetic names into a phonetic code.

Name	Phonetic Code
1. Chase, Vivian	_____
2. DeGrotte, Alma	_____
3. Gjerdahl, Felicia R	_____
4. Kollar, Rosa	_____
5. Schrader, Laurie	_____
6. Toutloff, Andrew	_____
7. Whittington, Lee	_____

See page 74 for answers.

Student Name _____

Check Your Knowledge

Directions:

For each of the items, circle the letter of the correct response.

Example:

0. The key indexing unit in the name Lloyd M. Charles is

    a. Lloyd

    (b.) Charles

    c. M

1. Which of the following names would be filed first?

    a. A. J. Chandler

    b. Aaron J. Chandler

    c. A. James Chandler

    d. Ai-lien Chandler

2. Which of the following names would be filed last?

    a. Brother Mark

    b. M. B. Brother

    c. Mark B. Brother

    d. Brother Mark Benson

3. Which of the following names would be filed second?

    a. Joseph M. Gerzin, Junior

    b. Joseph M. Gerzin, Sr.

    c. Joseph M. Gerzin, II

4. What is the second indexing unit in the name Dr. Clyde St. John?

    a. Clyde

    b. Saint

    c. St. John

5. Professional titles such as Dr. are indexed as what unit?

    a. first unit

    b. not indexed

    c. last unit

6. Miss Sara M. Ives is filed immediately before

    a. Judge Julio Mc Iver

    b. Juanita Mac Iver, MD

    c. Professor Jana Mc Ives

7. Which name would be filed third?

    a. Yoko O. Mori, Warsaw, IN

    b. Yoko O. Mori, Warsaw, IL

    c. Yoko O. Mori, Warsaw, ID

8. George Ellis Van de Hamme is filed before

    a. Liza de la Croix

    b. Kurt Van der Hamme

    c. Chris P. Van Haus

9. The name Jos. W. Small would be filed after

    a. J. W. Small

    b. Joseph Wm. Small

    c. Joe W. Small

10. The name that is filed last is

    a. Leonor Ester Sanchez

    b. Leon Eduardo Sanchez

    c. Gloria B. Rios-Sanchez

    d. Virginia M. Reyes-Sanchez

11. In phonetic filing, which is the primary code letter in Claude Martin?

    a.   the letter m

    b.   the letter c

    c.   there are only code numbers

12. In phonetic filing, which of the letters will be assigned a code number in the name Robbie McDitman?

    a.   m, c, t

    b.   c, d, m

    c.   c, d, t

Apply Your Knowledge of Alphabetic Filing

Directions:

Tear out the 30 alphabetic cards on page 89 and arrange them in alphabetic order following the alphabetic rules in Unit 2. After the cards are arranged in alphabetic order, write the names on the filing answer sheet on page 28 in the order in which you arranged the cards. Write the names in the order of indexing.

Example: Dr. Jorge J. Mier

MIER   JORGE   J   DR

Student Name _____

Apply Your Knowledge Alphabetic Filing
Answer Sheet

1. _____   16. _____

2. _____   17. _____

3. _____   18. _____

4. _____   19. _____

5. _____   20. _____

6. _____   21. _____

7. _____   22. _____

8. _____   23. _____

9. _____   24. _____

10. _____   25. _____

11. _____   26. _____

12. _____   27. _____

13. _____   28. _____

14. _____   29. _____

15. _____   30. _____

Unit 3

Numeric Filing

Objectives

After completing this unit, you will be able to:

1. Describe serial, unit, serial-unit, and social security numbering systems.

2. Describe the procedure for storing records by consecutive numeric, terminal-digit, and middle-digit filing methods.

3. File numeric cards in consecutive, terminal-digit, and middle-digit order.

As its name suggests, the numeric method of records storage is storage where records are assigned numbers and then stored in one of various numeric sequences. Two major reasons for using a numeric storage method are the ease with which people recognize and use numbers and the infinite set of numbers available.

FILING MEDICAL RECORDS BY NUMBER

The numeric filing method is used frequently when filing medical records, especially in large health care facilities. Each patient is assigned a number, and the medical records are filed by that number. A numeric filing system maintains the confidentiality of medical records as the number on the tab of the folder does not reveal the identity of a patient. In numeric filing, an accession ledger and patient card file (also known as the master patient index) are necessary for assignment of numbers and retrieval of medical records.

Accession Ledger

The **accession ledger** or book (sometimes known as a number logbook) contains a record of the consecutive numbers assigned to patients. The ledger provides (1) those numbers already assigned to patients and (2) the next number available for assignment. When a patient visits the medical facility, the next available number in the accession ledger is assigned to the patient, and the patient's name is written beside the number. (An accession ledger is shown in Figure 3.1.) This number identifies the patient and is written on all documents that refer to the patient. The patient folder contains the number, and is filed by this number. The accession ledger may be manual or computerized and is kept permanently.

Figure 3.1
Accession Ledger

#	File Name
ACCESSION LEDGER	
800	LAWSON, Sarah
801	SMITH, Fred
802	TREMONT Drug Supply
803	Mandelson, Trixie
804	
805	
808	
807	

Master Patient Index

A **master patient index** or patient card file contains an alphabetical listing of patients that is an essential cross-reference in numeric filing. The master patient index usually consists of 3- by 5-inch cards and is prepared after the patient's number is assigned. The patient card generally lists the patient's full name, address, telephone number, birth date, and patient number. Figure 3.2 shows a patient card. In retrieving a medical record filed numerically, the patient's card is located, and the patient number identified from the card. The patient medical record folder is then located in the file matching the number on the patient card file. The master patient index may also be computerized.

Figure 3.2
Patient Card

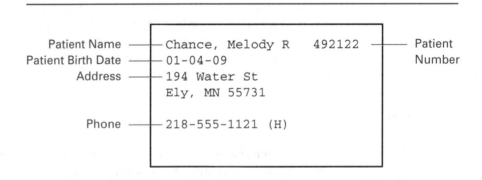

Patient Name ——— Chance, Melody R   492122 ——— Patient Number
Patient Birth Date ——— 01-04-09
Address ——— 194 Water St
Ely, MN 55731
Phone ——— 218-555-1121 (H)

Check Your Understanding

Directions:
Identify the sequence of steps to follow when assigning a patient number and when retrieving a medical record using numeric filing. Place the correct number in the space provided, with *1* indicating the first step and so on.

Assigning a Patient Number

_____ 1.   Prepare a patient card

_____ 2.   Enter patient name in accession book

_____ 3.   Write patient number on medical record

Retrieving a Medical Record

_____ 1.   Retrieve medical record from file

_____ 2.   Locate patient number on patient card

_____ 3.   Locate patient card in alphabetic card file

See page 74 for answers.

NUMBERING SYSTEMS

Numbers are assigned to patients to differentiate one patient from another. Health facilities will determine the numbering system that best meets their needs. Numbering systems include serial, unit, serial-unit, and social security numbers.

Serial Numbering

In **serial numbering,** the patient receives a new number at the time of each visit to a medical office or medical facility. The first time George Andrew is treated, he may receive the number 1122, the second time 1233, and so on. This means the medical records are filed in various places depending on the number of times a person visits. An advantage of serial numbering is that file expansion is not necessary as the thickness of the individual medical record does not change since a new record and folder are created at each visit. Also, previously assigned patient numbers do not need to be considered. A disadvantage is that continuity of care is lost unless all patient records are retrieved whenever a patient visits the medical facility. Also, retrieval and filing of numerous records for each patient is time-consuming. Serial numbering may be more suitable to hospitals without ambulatory care centers and is not recommended for physician's offices.

Unit Numbering

In **unit numbering,** the patient is assigned a patient number on the first visit and retains the same number for subsequent visits. With unit numbering, each time George Andrew visits, documentation of care will be under the same number. All medical records for a patient are filed in one place, which provides for continuity of care. A disadvantage is that medical records become thick with multiple visits, and more than one folder may be needed. Space must be allowed in the files for expansion, and from time to time it may be necessary to shift medical records to make more space. When unit numbering is utilized, it is also important to determine whether or not the patient has been previously assigned a number in order that a patient would not be assigned more than one number.

The use of a social security number may be adapted to unit numbering. A *social security number* is a unique identification number given to individuals by the Social Security Administration. An advantage of using a patient's social security number is that it is a number unique to that patient. Disadvantages are that the health care facility does not have control over the social security numbers and cannot verify numbers. In addition, some individuals may not have a social security number, and some may have more than one social security number. The medical facility would need to assign a "pseudo" social security number to those who do not have a social security number. Another disadvantage is there would be gaps in the shelf files as it is difficult to determine in advance what numbers patients would have. The Social Security Administration does not recommend use of social security numbers.

Serial-Unit Numbering

In **serial-unit numbering,** the patient receives a new number each time the patient visits. The previous medical records are brought forward and filed with the latest assigned number record. For example, Connie Lacy was issued number 94857 on her first visit. When she returns to the medical facility, number 98000 is assigned. Connie Lacy's medical record 94857 would be brought forward and filed with 98000 records. When older records are brought forward, the old folder or an OUT guide must be prepared and placed where the old chart was filed, indicating the new number. The advantage is that a unit record is created. A disadvantage is that records will need to be moved back as space is created when old records are moved forward.

FILING SYSTEMS

There are three types of numeric filing systems often used in medical facilities. They include consecutive numeric, terminal-digit, and middle-digit. The terminal-digit and middle-digit systems are nonconsecutive systems. This means that, for filing purposes, numbers are not read in their usual consecutive sequence from left to right.

Consecutive Numeric Filing

The **consecutive numeric filing** system is also known as straight numeric. It is the arrangement of medical records by assigned numbers, starting with the lowest number and ending with the highest. Numbers are read from left to right. The greatest advantage of using straight numeric filing is the ease of training personnel. Another advantage is that shelving units or other filing equipment can be added as storage becomes full. Disadvantages include the following: (1) the person filing medical records must consider all digits at one time, allowing for transposition of numbers, which may lead to misfiles; (2) work flow problems may develop, since ninety percent of file room activity will be centered in ten percent of the available space, that designated for the newest record numbers; and (3) as older medical records are purged, back shifting must be done.

The following numbers are arranged in consecutive numeric sequence. Notice that the numbers are arranged logically from smallest to largest.

458292
458295
459300
548000
548295

Check Your Understanding

Directions:
Arrange the following numbers in consecutive numeric order in the filing order column.

Consecutive Number	Filing Order
458731	1. _____
457813	2. _____
459313	3. _____
337021	4. _____
330712	5. _____
337012	6. _____
330172	7. _____

See page 74 for answers.

Terminal-Digit Filing

A **terminal digit** filing system groups numbers into units containing two digits each. Usually a six-digit number is used and divided with a hyphen into three parts. The digits are read from right to left. The last two digits of a number are the first indexing unit and are called *primary digits*. The *secondary digits* are the middle two digits and are the second indexing unit. The *tertiary digits* are the first two digits and are the third indexing unit.

Number	Tertiary Digits	Secondary Digits	Primary Digits
12-32-44	12	32	44
13-33-45	13	33	45
13-43-45	13	43	45

In a terminal-digit file, there are 100 primary sections ranging from 00 to 99. The medical record is first taken to the primary section corresponding to its terminal digits. Within the primary section, groups of medical records are matched according to secondary digits. After locating the appropriate secondary section, the medical record is filed within it in numeric order by the tertiary digits. In the file, the tertiary digit changes with every medical record. For example, for 45-22-02 the filing location is first narrowed to the primary section 02, then the secondary section 22, then the tertiary position 45.

Sequence in a Terminal-Digit File

Numbers in Sequence	Primary Digits	Secondary Digits	Tertiary Digits
45-22-02	02	22	45
46-22-02	02	22	46
47-22-02	02	22	47

Figure 3.3 shows an example of terminal-digit filing in the file area.

Terminal-digit filing normally involves six digits but can be adapted for use with any number of digits. If five digits are used, they would be divided as 1-21-22. If seven digits are used, they would be divided as 332-33-22; and if four digits are used, they would be divided as 22-42. The advantage of terminal-digit filing is that the individual filing the medical records does not need to remember several digits at a time, which will reduce the chances of transposing numbers, thus reducing misfiles. Another advantage is that medical records can be presorted by primary numbers, and several individuals may file at the same time without crowding the file area. A disadvantage is that more training time may be required than with straight numeric filing. Expansion of the total file area must be planned for from the start, and sufficient shelf files or other storage equipment must be purchased. Space in the files must be left to accommodate the patient records as they are filed by terminal digit. Terminal-digit filing was developed to make numeric filing and retrieval more efficient and accurate.

Check Your Understanding

Directions:
Rearrange the following numbers into correct terminal-digit filing order. The first is an example as to how the number should be written.

Numbers		Terminal-Digit Filing Order
12-35-81	1.	36-34-18
13-35-81	2.	_____
23-43-18	3.	_____
36-34-18	4.	_____

23-44-18   5. _____

24-44-18   6. _____

23-43-81   7. _____

35-34-81   8. _____

See page 74 for answers.

Middle-Digit Filing

In **middle-digit filing,** numbers are grouped according to pairs of digits as in terminal-digit filing. However, primary numbers are the middle two digits of a six digit number, secondary numbers are the first two numbers, and tertiary numbers are the last two digits of a number.

Sequence in a Middle-Digit File

Numbers in Sequence	Primary Digits	Secondary Digits	Tertiary Digits
23-48-91	48	23	91
23-50-91	50	23	91
23-50-92	50	23	92

As with terminal-digit filing, middle-digit filing is by pairs of digits; therefore reducing misfiles. Middle-digit filing is more complicated, and training time of personnel is more extensive than with consecutive and terminal-digit filing. Middle-digit filing does not lend itself to numbers with more than six digits.

Check Your Understanding

Directions:
Rearrange the following numbers into correct middle-digit filing order. The first one has been inserted as an example as how the numbers should be written.

Numbers		Middle-Digit Filing Order
32-89-57	1.	23-89-56
32-89-56	2.	_____
23-89-56	3.	_____
23-92-56	4.	_____
23-92-50	5.	_____
23-92-51	6.	_____
24-93-56	7.	_____
32-92-56	8.	_____

See page 75 for answers.

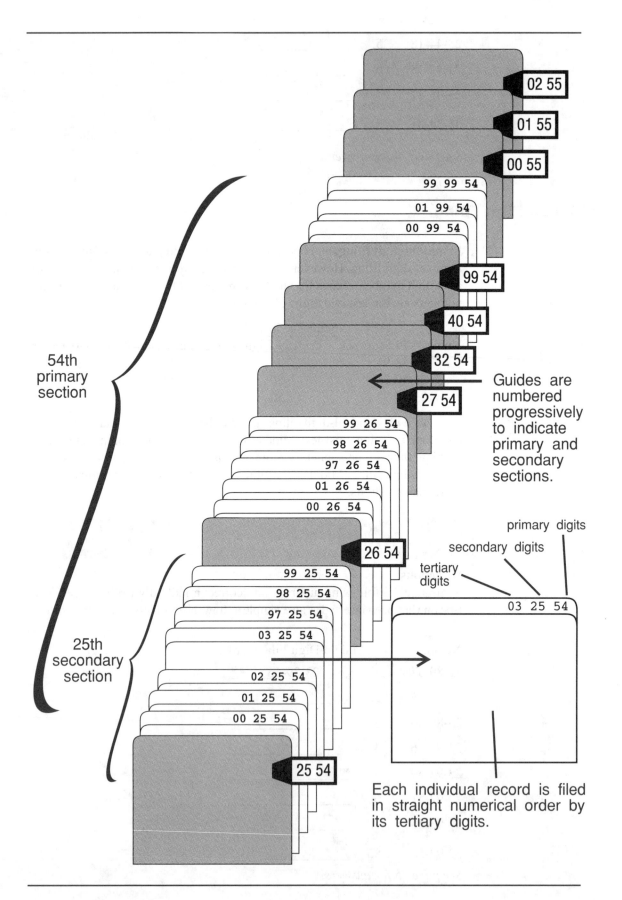

02 55

01 55

00 55

99 99 54

01 99 54

00 99 54

99 54

40 54

32 54

Guides are
numbered
progressively
to indicate
primary and
secondary
sections.

27 54

99 26 54

98 26 54

97 26 54

01 26 54

00 26 54

54th
primary
section

primary digits

secondary digits

tertiary
digits

26 54

99 25 54

98 25 54

97 25 54

03 25 54

25th
secondary
section

03 25 54

02 25 54

01 25 54

00 25 54

25 54

Each individual record is filed
in straight numerical order by
its tertiary digits.

Figure 3.3   Terminal-Digit Filing

Student Name _____

Check Your Knowledge

Directions:
In the space provided to the left of Column A, write the letter of the term in Column B that fits the definition.

Column A

_____ 1. Filing medical records by number rather than by letter.

_____ 2. A cross-reference for numeric filing.

_____ 3. Numbering system in which the patient retains the same number for all visits.

_____ 4. A list of the numbers assigned to patients when numeric filing is used.

_____ 5. Simplest numeric filing method in terms of training personnel.

_____ 6. Numeric filing system in which 64 in the number 456412 is the secondary unit.

_____ 7. Numeric filing system that must have six digits.

_____ 8. A patient is assigned a new number on each visit in this numbering system.

_____ 9. The third indexing unit in terminal-digit and middle-digit filing.

_____ 10. The first indexing unit in terminal-digit or middle-digit filing.

Column B

A.   accession ledger

B.   terminal-digit

C.   tertiary

D.   numeric

E.   unit

F.   middle-digit

G.   serial

H.   consecutive or straight

I.   patient card

J.   primary

Apply Your Knowledge of Numeric Filing

Directions:

Tear out the thirty numeric cards starting on page 89 and arrange them in consecutive numeric order. After the cards are arranged in consecutive numeric order, write the consecutive numbers on the numeric answer sheet on page 40 in the order in which you arranged the cards. After you have completed the consecutive numeric filing, do the same for terminal-digit and middle-digit filing. The answers to the first one have been inserted as an example as to how the numbers should be written.

Student Name

Apply Your Knowledge Numeric Filing Answer

	Consecutive	Terminal-Digit	Middle-Digit
1.	8015	21-00-15	05-00-75
2.			
3.			
4.			
5.			
6.			
7.			
8.			
9.			
10.			
11.			
12.			
13.			
14.			
15.			
16.			
17.			
18.			
19.			
20.			
21.			
22.			
23.			
24.			
25.			
26.			
27.			
28.			
29			
30.			

Unit 4

Cross-Referencing

Objectives

After completing this unit, you will be able to:

1. Identify the purpose of cross-referencing.

2. Identify four types of personal names that require cross-referencing and give an example of each.

3. Cross-reference personal names.

4. Describe cross-referencing in numeric filing.

While filing medical records, it may be necessary to use cross-referencing for retrieval of medical records. Cross-referencing is a means by which a notation is made in one location to indicate that the medical record or master patient index card may be stored elsewhere. In alphabetic filing, medical records are filed under the name most likely to be requested. Other possible names are considered, and a cross-reference is created directing personnel to where the medical record file is located. In numeric filing, an alphabetic card file is used for cross-referencing the patient name and number. It may also be necessary to cross-reference numbers on the medical records if for some reason the patient number should change. While cross-referencing assists in location of medical record files, it must be used with discretion. Each cross-reference requires additional paper to be stored, which is not only costly and time-consuming but also takes more space.

ALPHABETIC CROSS-REFERENCING

Alphabetic cross-referencing is used when a name might be indexed in more than one way. It may be used for unusual, alternate, hyphenated, and similar names.

Unusual Names

In unusual names, the last name may be difficult to determine or unfamiliar, such as in foreign names. When determining the last name is difficult, index the last name first on the original medical record and prepare a cross-reference with the first name indexed first. Thomas Gregory would be filed under GREGORY

THOMAS, and a cross-reference would be prepared under THOMAS GREGORY with a notation to see GREGORY THOMAS. Other examples of unusual names are George Lloyd, Lu Liu, and Bernard Franklin.

Table 4.1

Original Medical File	Cross-Reference Card
LLOYD GEORGE	GEORGE LLOYD SEE LLOYD GEORGE
LIU LU	LU LIU SEE LIU LU
FRANKLIN BERNARD	BERNARD FRANKLIN SEE FRANKLIN BERNARD

Alternate Names

Sometimes a patient goes by more than one name or changes names. Some reasons for alternate names are use of a married name, a husband's first name, or a professional name. Other reasons include a name change as a result of being adopted or returning to a maiden name. Examples of alternate names are Mrs. Janice Lynn Market and Mrs. James Market, Clara Iris Lopez and Mrs. Clara Iris Perez, William John Layman and Bill Layman, Joseph Hiermstad and Joey Herman, Amy C. Kelly and Amy C. Simpson, Cathy Klein and Cathy Rosenbaun.

Table 4.2

Original Medical File	Cross-Reference Card	Reason for Alternate Name
MARKET JANICE LYNN	MARKET JAMES MRS SEE MARKET JANICE LYNN	Husband's name
LOPEZ CLARA IRIS	PEREZ CLARA IRIS (MRS) SEE LOPEZ CLARA IRIS	Married name
LAYMAN WILLIAM JOHN	LAYMAN BILL SEE LAYMAN WILLIAM JOHN	Nickname
HJERMSTAD JOSEPH	HERMAN JOEY SEE HJERMSTAD JOSEPH	Professional name
KELLY AMY C	SIMPSON AMY C SEE KELLY AMY C	Return to maiden name
KLIEN CATHY	ROESENBAUN CATHY SEE KLIEN CATHY	Adoption by stepfather

Hyphenated Names

In indexing hyphenated names, the hyphen is disregarded. It may be confusing or difficult to determine the last name if the hyphen is left out of the name and the names separated. Examples of hyphenated surnames are Mary P. Winter-White, Nam Rice-Ling, and L. R. Benson-Smith.

Table 4.3

Original Medical File	Cross-Reference Card
WINTERWHITE MARY P	WHITE MARY P WINTER SEE WINTERWHITE MARY P
RICELING NAM	LING NAM RICE SEE RICELING NAM
BENSONSMITH L R	SMITH L R BENSON SEE BENSONSMITH L R

Similar Names

Names that sound alike but are spelled differently are known as similar names. *See also* cross-references are prepared for all possible spellings. An example is the name Maki, which may also be spelled Macke or Mackey.

Table 4.4

Cross-Reference Card

MAKI	MACKEY	MACKE
SEE ALSO MACKEY MACKE	SEE ALSO MAKI MACKE	SEE ALSO MAKI MACKEY
MCGEE	MAGEE	
SEE ALSO MAGEE	SE ALSO MCGEE	
MAAS	MOSS	
SEE ALSO MOSS	SEE ALSO MAAS	

Check Your Understanding

Directions:

Below are five names to be cross-referenced. Write the primary form of indexing under the name. On the right, write the name for cross-referencing with the reference back to the original.

Example:

0. John Stephen   JOHN STEPHEN
    STEPHEN JOHN   SEE: STEPHEN JOHN

1. Anna Maria Lacy (Mrs. Bill)   _____

    _____   SEE: _____

2. Sheng Tien   _____

    _____   SEE: _____

3. Iola Hansen
    (could be spelled Hanson)   _____

    _____   SEE: _____

4. Carrie Nicholas-Hans   _____

    _____   SEE: _____

5. George Thomas   _____

    _____   SEE: _____

See page 75 for answers.

NUMERIC CROSS-REFERENCING

Cross-referencing is necessary when medical records are filed numerically. The patient's alphabetic card would contain the number under which the medical record is filed. Before a medical record can be retrieved, the patient card would first be located, the number on the card determined, and then the medical record retrieved. See Figure 4.1, a patient card with numeric cross-referencing.

Figure 4.1
Cross-Reference
for Numeric Filing

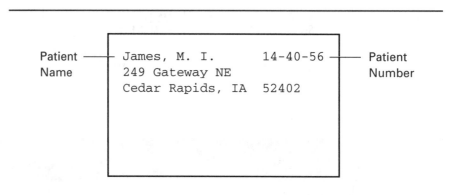

Patient Name — James, M. I.   14-40-56 — Patient Number
249 Gateway NE
Cedar Rapids, IA   52402

Numeric cross-referencing is also necessary if a patient number changes. This may occur when a medical facility converts numbering systems. When a patient visits the medical facility after the conversion to a new numbering system, a new number is assigned, and the previous medical files are brought forward to the new file. A cross-reference is placed in the previous file indicating the new file number. Cross-referencing is also used in serial-unit numbering systems. In serial-unit numbering the patient is assigned a new number on each visit, and the previous file is brought forward.

Student Name _____

Check Your Knowledge

Directions:
For each name below, indicate the name under which the primary medical record would be filed and the name under which the record would be cross-referenced. Numbers 3 and 12 will require two cross-references each. The first one is done as an example.

Name	Primary Medical File	Cross-Reference
0. Sally Lane (Mrs. J. R.)	LANE SALLY	LANE J R MRS
1. An Wang	_____	_____
2. George David	_____	_____
3. Irene Sylvester (marries Robert K. Brooks)	_____	_____
		_____
4. Veronica K. Larson (could be spelled Larsen)	_____	_____
5. Lamonte Roach (a musician using the name Lanny Lamonte professionally)	_____	_____
6. Carol Rose-Braun	_____	_____
7. Katherine Stark (uses her maiden name Katherine Lester)	_____	_____
8. Rinji Akita	_____	_____
9. Melissa Cruz (adopted by Allen B. Wade)	_____	_____
10. Gerald Z. Von Yeast (called Jerry Von Yeast)	_____	_____
11. Jeanine Vick (husband's first name is Addison)	_____	_____
12. Angelica Jensen (marries Raymond Rivera)	_____	_____
		_____
13. Ismael Martinez (also known as Mike Martinez)	_____	_____
14. Kim Rose	_____	_____
15. Jane Livingston-Ramos	_____	_____

Unit 5

Color Coding

Objectives

After completing this unit, you will be able to:

1. Identify the purpose of color coding for medical records filing.

2. Identify the two numeric filing systems that are best suited for color coding.

3. Identify two areas other than alphabetic and numeric filing where color coding may be utilized.

4. Describe alphabetic color coding.

5. Describe numeric color coding.

6. Identify how misfiles are recognized in color-coded medical files.

In many medical filing systems, colors are used on medical records folders to provide personnel with a way to file and retrieve medical records quickly. This method not only makes filing more efficient but also helps to reduce misfiles. In **color-coded filing systems,** a color is assigned to each letter (in alphabetic filing) or number (in numeric filing). The colors are then used to mark each file folder. For example, in alphabetic filing, colors might be used to indicate the first two letters of the patient's last name. The colors are placed in predetermined positions on the file folder. Color bars or patterns in various positions create large patterns of colored blocks in file drawers or on shelves. A break in the color pattern will signal a misfiled medical record. Color coding simplifies auditing or checking the files for misfiled records.

Commercial color-coded folders may be purchased with preprinted color-coded letters or numbers; or a medical facility can create their own by use of self-adhesive color-coded labels on plain folders.

Color coding was originally developed as part of terminal-digit filing but may also be used to signify information not associated with filing. The file folder may indicate the last year a patient was seen in a medical facility by displaying a color assigned to that year. Color coding the year a patient last visited would assist in the identification of inactive medical records. For example, if a red label is assigned to the year 1988, and all medical records are considered inactive if a patient has not visited for three years, then in 1992 personnel could readily locate the red year stickers and remove the medical records from the active file. These inactive records could be destroyed, microfilmed, or moved to inactive storage. Another use may be to indicate the patient's primary physician.

ALPHABETIC COLOR CODING

In alphabetic color coding, a color scheme is used to identify letters of the alphabet. Figure 5.1 shows a partial color code chart for alphabetic letters.

Figure 5.1
Partial Alphabetic
Color Coding Chart

Letter Represented	Color
A	Brown
B	Yellow
C	Orange
D	Light Blue
E	Blue
F	Pink
G	Green
H	White
I	Grey
J	Red

Combinations of letters will form color patterns. There are various methods of color coding letters for filing. One way to color code letters is to color code the first two letters of a patient's last name. For example, in the name Jensen, *J* is represented by red and *e* by blue. Folders for all patients whose names start with *Je* show red and blue. Figure 5.2 shows color coding of folders for alphabetic filing.

In the first position is the primary guide, which divides the alphabet. This letter is color-coded. For instance, all folders for names beginning with *J* will be red in the first position. Personnel will be able to identify the main alphabetic file section with the color red when filing medical files with last names beginning with *J*. Position two contains the patient's full name. The third and fourth positions contain the first two letters of the patient's last name (*J* and *e* in the name Jensen) and are color-coded. After filing the first two letters of the last the name in the color-coded area, the medical record will be filed by the rest of the name according to alphabetic rules you learned in Unit 2. For example, Jensen will be filed before Jepson.

When a medical record file shows the color red and brown in the third and fourth positions, it represents *Ja*. If this medical record is filed with the *Je* section, a misfile would be readily noted as the color pattern would be broken. Figure 5.3 shows two misfiled records, apparent by a break in the color pattern.

Figure 5.2
Color Coding
for Alphabetic Filing

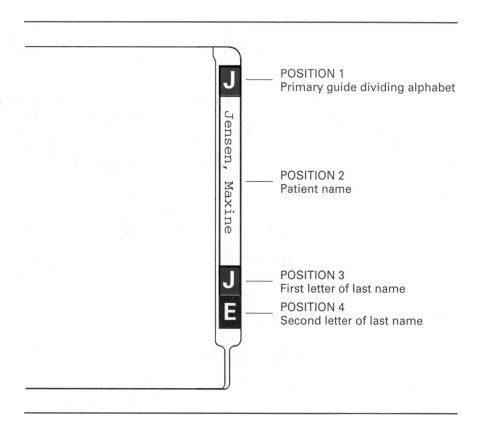

POSITION 1
Primary guide dividing alphabet

POSITION 2
Patient name

POSITION 3
First letter of last name

POSITION 4
Second letter of last name

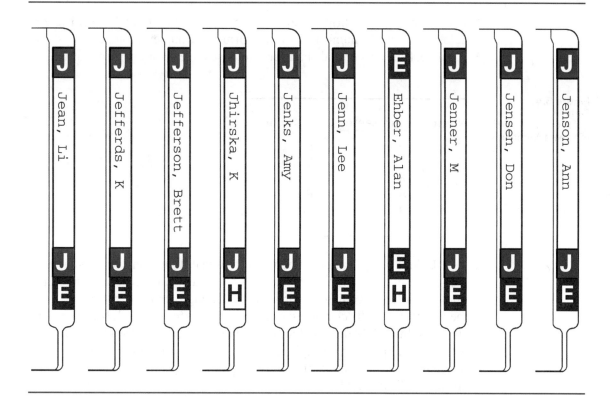

Figure 5.3 Color-Coded Alphabetic File

Check Your Understanding

Directions:

Using the color code chart in Figure 5.1, determine the color coding scheme for each of the following names. The first one is done as an example.

	Name	Color Scheme Position 3	Position 4
0.	Bud B. Jensen	red	blue
1.	Ramos Hewitt	_____	_____
2.	Carlos A. Gaffey	_____	_____
3.	Jamie Diaz	_____	_____
4.	Miss Sandra Garcia	_____	_____
5.	Dr. Renee Benton-Jenkins	_____	_____

See page 75 for answers.

NUMERIC COLOR CODING

In the same way that different colors represent letters of the alphabet, different colors represent the numbers zero through nine in a numeric color code system. Figure 5.4 shows a partial chart for a color scheme for numeric coding.

Figure 5.4
Partial
Color Coding Chart
of Patient Numbers

Number Represented	Color
0	Pink
1	White
6	Blue
8	Red
9	Light Blue

Color coding is most effective in terminal-digit filing or middle-digit filing. However, it can be made workable for straight numeric filing. In setting up numeric color coding, all or some of the digits may be color-coded. A medical facility will determine the number of digits to color code based on their situation. In middle-digit and terminal-digit filing, two color blocks or bars appear in each position signifying primary, secondary, or tertiary digits. Figure 5.5 shows how the number 01-10-61 in terminal-digit filing would be color-coded for all six digits.

Color coding only the primary digits is known as two-band color coding. When four-band color coding is used, the primary and secondary digits are

Figure 5.5
Color Coding for
Terminal-Digit Filing

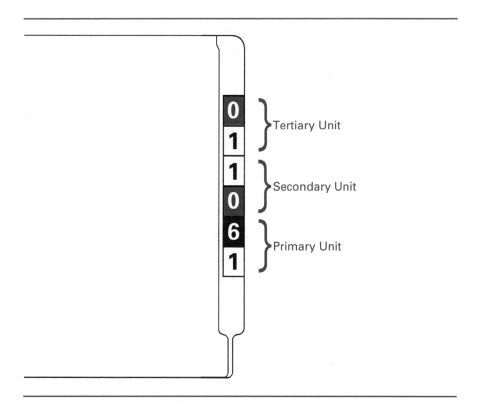

color-coded. In six-band coding, all digits are color-coded. Sometimes only three digits are color-coded. If all the patient numbers are not color-coded, the remaining numbers are written on the medical file folder in order to identify the patient record. A break in the color pattern will signify a misfile. Figure 5.6 shows three-band numeric color coding with two misfiled records.

Figure 5.6
Color Coded
Numeric Filing

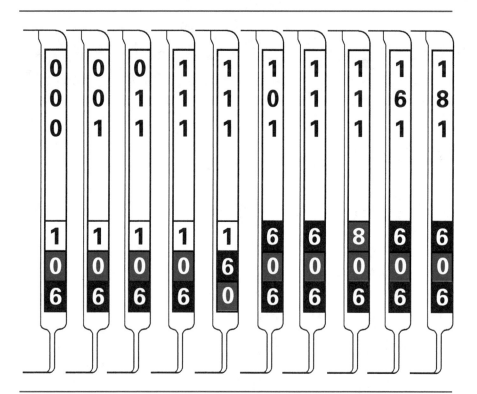

Check Your Understanding

Directions:
Using the color code chart in Figure 5.4, determine the color coding scheme for each of the following numbers. The first one is done as an example.

	Number	Color Scheme		
		Primary	Secondary	Tertiary
0.	01-66-06	pink-blue	blue-blue	pink-white
1.	01-98-06	_____	_____	_____
2.	01-99-06	_____	_____	_____
3.	01-89-08	_____	_____	_____
4.	06-11-09	_____	_____	_____
5.	08-10-90	_____	_____	_____

See page 75 for answers.

Student Name _____

Check Your Knowledge

Directions:
Respond to each of the following items with a short answer.

1. Identify the purpose of color coding.

   _____

2. Identify two items of information that may be color-coded on medical records files in addition to patient names and numbers.

   _____

3. Describe how personnel may identify misfiles with color-coded medical records files.

   _____

4. Using the color code system described in *Medical Filing,* which letters of a patient's name are color-coded?

   _____

5. Identify the two types of numeric filing best suited to color coding.

   _____

6. For the terminal-digit number 01-09-99, describe how the tab on the medical records file folder would be color-coded using four-band color coding according to the color coding scheme in *Medical Filing.*

   _____

7. Color code the patient name file for the name Gabriel Fenton, using the color code in *Medical Filing.*

   _____

8. Color coding medical records files eliminates misfiles. Is this statement true or false?

   _____

9. Identify the purpose of color coding the year the patient was last seen at a medical facility.

   _____

10. To quickly file the medical record of Johann Abernathy, identify the steps you would go through in a color-coded filing system.

    _____

This exercise continues on the following page.

11. Describe how to audit or check the *De* section of the file area using color codes.

_____

12. Describe how to quickly audit or check the primary section 06 in color-coded terminal-digit filing.

_____

Apply Your Knowledge of Color Coding

Directions:
Follow the steps below to apply your knowledge of color coding.

1.   File the 30 color-coded cards on page 87 in the following order.

Filing Order

1. Julia Delgado	16. Dick Fharger
2. Rev. Johnnie Deppe	17. Reva M. Feuss
3. Lumir Djerk	18. Clarence Doc Fewell
4. Virgil L. Derby	19. Juan Feye
5. M. Louise Dergo	20. Angelique Hearn
6. MarJoan Edgar	21. Yoko S. Heath
7. Waldo Edleman	22. Olivia Heathman
8. Louis Edlin, M.D.	23. Miss Emma Hjemboe
9. Ms. Kim Edmond	24. Judge Benji Hebel
10. Brother Gerald Eeckhoff	25. Ching-Yu Heck
11. Thomas G. Eells	26. E.L. Hjermstad
12. Sister LuAnn Edward	27. Amelia S. Heidt
13. Lin Feng	28. Marcus P. Jeanblanc
14. Ms. Hazel Fernandenz	29. Scott P. Jehle
15. Carlos Fetzer	30. Thomas A. Jewell

2.   After the cards are filed, identify any misfiles in the alphabetic order by a break in the color pattern for letters.

3.   On the answer sheet on page 56 list the names that were filed incorrectly.

4.   After writing the patient names that were misfiled, refile the cards in correct alphabetic order. Double-check your work for misfiles by checking the color pattern.

5.   At this point the cards are arranged correctly for alphabetic filing but not for numeric filing. If these thirty cards are to be filed using the terminal-digit method, which ones are misfiled? List the entire number for each misfiled card. Be sure to write the numbers as it appears on the card-tertiary, secondary, primary.

6.   Correctly refile the misfiled numeric cards and double-check your filing by checking the color patterns.

Student Name
_____

Apply Your Knowledge Color Coding
Answer Sheet

Alphabetic Misfiled Cards

1. _____

2. _____

3. _____

4 _____

5. _____

Numeric Misfiled Cards

1. _____

2. _____

3. _____

4 _____

5. _____

6. _____

Unit 6

Records Control

Objectives

After completing this unit, you will be able to:

1. Discuss the purpose of charge-out procedures when a medical record is borrowed.

2. Identify three advantages of an automated tracking system.

3. List four questions to be considered before medical records are transferred and possible answers.

4. Describe the difference between active and inactive medical records and indicate how each is determined.

5. Specify the recommended time period medical records should be retained.

6. Describe appropriate methods for destruction of medical records.

Records control refers to procedures used to keep track of medical records once they have been created. If no records control procedures exist, medical records will not be easily located. If medical records are not available when needed, continuity of care becomes difficult. Also, unnecessary time will be spent trying to locate the medical records. It is necessary for a medical facility to develop policies and procedures for charging out medical records, for identifying what constitutes an active or inactive medical record, for determining how long medical records should be retained, and for transferring records. It is recommended that a single individual be responsible for developing policies and procedures and training employees in records control methods. Without policies and procedures and proper training, a medical record may find its way to unauthorized personnel. This could result in loss of confidentiality of information on the part of the patient and possible litigation against the medical facility. If the medical record cannot be located for use as a reference when caring for the patient, unnecessary treatments may occur. Sometimes this is harmful to the patient, and once again litigation against the medical facility may result. Consistency is the key to good records control.

CHARGE-OUT PROCEDURES

Charge-out procedures assure that all medical records are accounted for and that the borrower is responsible for returning the medical record to the storage area for filing. Charge-out procedures should be followed regardless of who removes the medical record from the files, for what reason, or for how long. Less than one minute is needed to note the borrower of the medical record, while hours can be spent searching for lost or misplaced medical records. A charge-out system generally consists of requisition, OUT guide and follow-up mechanism.

Requisitions

A **requisition** is a request for a medical record. The request may be made by telephone, mail, or in person and is put in writing by the requestor or by records personnel. Such a written request is known as a *requisition form*. Information on the requisition form includes name of patient, medical record number if applicable, borrower's name, location where record is to be taken, date removed from the file, and date to be returned. Figure 6.1 shows a requisition form.

Figure 6.1
Requisition Form

```
REQUISITION FOR MEDICAL RECORDS

Patient's Name_____

Record Number_____

Date Taken_____

Date To Be Returned_____

Location_____

Requested By_____
```

The requisition form may be a three-part form. One copy is placed in the file from which the medical record is removed, one is fastened to the medical record, and one is maintained in a tickler file. A **tickler file** serves as a reminder that specific action is to be taken on a specific date. Requisition forms are arranged in the tickler file according to the date medical records are to be returned. When the medical records are returned, the requisition in the tickler file is removed. If medical records are not returned by the specified date, the tickler file serves as a ready reference to identify overdue medical records and remind the borrower to return the record. If a tickler file is not used, personnel would need to check the files on a routine basis to identify records that have been out longer than the specified time. When requisition forms are used, it is important to have the entire form completed, regardless of the reason for removal of the medical record.

OUT Guides

An OUT guide is a special guide used to replace any medical record removed from the file and remains in the file until the medical record is returned. Use of an OUT guide provides a means for record control. OUT guides should be of sturdy construction since they are reused many times. They may contain a pocket at the front for the requisition form or have a cumulative guide on which information can be written.

Either type of OUT guide will provide information as to the exact location of the medical record if personnel are trying to locate a record that is not in the file. Figure 6.2 shows the two types of OUT guides.

Figure 6.2
Two Types
of OUT Guides

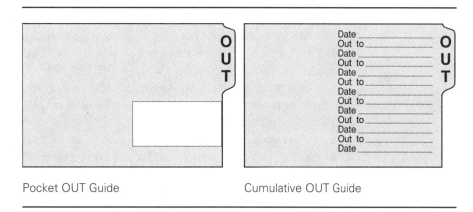

Pocket OUT Guide   Cumulative OUT Guide

OUT guides may be colored. Colored OUT guides are helpful in spotting the location of medical records for refiling. However, personnel must check to be sure the medical record is being returned to the proper location. Different colored guides may also be used for different weeks or days, which would assist in determining which medical records have been out for what period of time. In a medical clinic where there is more than one physician, a color could be designated for each physician, which again would assist in determining where a medical record is located. An OUT guide is to be placed in the file whenever a medical record is removed and a notation made of the location of the record. The few minutes personnel take to note the location of the record and insert the OUT guide where it was removed may save a great deal of time later searching for it.

Follow-Up Procedures

Follow-up is checking on the return of borrowed medical records within a reasonable length of time. The length of time medical records may be out of the file is determined by the needs of the medical facility and the number of requests. A time limit should be established, and procedures for follow-up of overdue medical records should be implemented. The longer medical records remain out of the files, the more difficult the return becomes as they may become misplaced; thus, two weeks is the maximum time recommended for records to be borrowed.

When a requisition form is used, a copy may be placed in a tickler file under the due date. When the medical record is returned, the requisition form is removed from the tickler file, the medical record is returned to the file and the OUT guide is removed. If a tickler file is not used, personnel must check the OUT guides in the files on a routine basis to identify records that have been out longer than the specified time. When medical records are not returned by the due date, personnel will use a follow-up method to identify the borrowers and then contact them for return of the medical records.

AUTOMATED TRACKING SYSTEM

An **automated tracking system** provides information on location of medical records at any given point in time using a computer. The system may utilize a stand alone microcomputer or may interface with the mainframe information system. In order to sign out a medical record, the stand alone microcomputer requires inputting the patient name, medical record number, and location of medical record. The computer will automatically record date and time of each transaction. If the tracking system interfaces with the master patient index either the patient name or medical record will be entered and also the required check out information.

Bar codes representing patient numbers which are printed on the folder of the medical record may also be used to speed up the process. Bar codes resemble those found on merchandise in stores and are scanned in a similar way. A bar code reader consists of a small computer terminal with a wand to read the bar codes. The identification of the medical record is recorded and the remaining information required to complete the charge out transaction is entered via a keyboard. The automated tracking system generates sign out slips for outguides. Figure 6.3 shows a computer generated sign out slip.

Figure 6.3
Computer Charge
Out Slip

Patient Name: Yoko S. Heath		Medical Number: 19-08-68	
Dated Pulled	**Old Location**	**New Location**	**Telephone**
3/21/96	Medical Records	Dr. K. Frank	4111
Dated Requested	Time Requested		
3/20/96	4:00PM		

The automated tracking system also creates lists of pending requests which will assist in pulling medical records in a timely manner, return reminder lists for medical records kept past the designated time, and will show past activity and the location of each medical record. An example of current and past activity and the location of a patient's medical record is shown in Figure 6.4.

Advantages of automated record tracking system are that it improves record access, facilitates record retrieval, and reduces the incidence of misplaced medical records.

Figure 6.4
Medical Record
Activity and Location

Patient Name: Maria Lopez   **Medical Record Number: 22-33-69**

<u>CURRENT LOCATION</u>

Requester:	Date	Time	Location	Telephone
R. Johans	4/14/96	10:00AM	X-ray	4389

<u>PREVIOUS LOCATION</u>

Requester	Date	Time	Location	Telephone
R. Cram	3/15/96	1:00PM	Insurance	4444
Dr. DeNarr	3/1/96	9:00AM	Office	4400
T. Miller	3/1/96	10:00AM	X-ray	4436
M. Ichen	3/1/96	10:15AM	Lab	4442

Check Your Understanding

Directions:
In the space provided, fill in the term that fits the definition or question.

1. Checking on the return of medical records within a reasonable length of time.

   _____

2. A form containing information on the location of a medical record removed from the files.

   _____

3. A card placed in the file when a medical record is removed.

   _____

4. Personnel do not need to indicate when a medical record is being borrowed for less than a day. Is this statement true or false?

   _____

5. A file that specifies the date on which borrowed medical records are to be returned.

   _____

6. Automated tracking system must use a Bar Code. Is this true or false?

   _____

7. List the three advantages of an automated chart tracking system.

   _____

   _____

   _____

See page 74 for answers.

RETENTION AND DESTRUCTION OF MEDICAL RECORDS

The length of time medical records should be kept depends on the health facility needs, existing state laws, and potential for litigation. Not all states have laws designating how long medical records should be retained. Retention of medical records may be determined by a statute of limitations. A **statute of limitations** specifies the time frame for bringing legal action. In most states this time period is less than ten years for injury or breach of contract. Many states also have a statute of limitations for minors specifying that legal action for personal injuries must be initiated within two to three years after the minor has attained legal age. Medical records that are more than ten years old are seldom requested from a health care facility for legal, clinical, or scientific purposes. In the absence of state law, it is usually sufficient to maintain medical records for ten years after the most recent patient care episode. The American Health Information Management Association and American Hospital Association recommend ten years for retention of medical records if there is no state statute.

Unless destruction is prohibited by law, medical records to be destroyed should be burned or shredded to assure confidentiality. If medical records are destroyed, the health care facility must retain basic information such as diagnoses, procedures, dates of treatment, and responsible physician. Health care facilities may wish to consider alternate means of storage, such as microfilming, optical or magnetic disk storage, or computer patient records rather than destruction of medical records. These alternate storage methods were discussed in Unit 1. Cost will be a consideration when determining whether or not alternate storage methods are utilized. Each health facility should establish policies for retention and destruction of medical records with the assistance of their legal counsel and liability insurance carrier.

TRANSFER PROCEDURES

Once medical records are stored in the file area, they do not stay there forever. It may be necessary to transfer some medical records to another area to make room for more current medical records. In identifying medical records for transfer, those that are not used frequently will be selected. Four questions must be answered before transferring of medical records can take place:

- WHAT medical records are to be moved?

- HOW will the medical records be prepared for transfer?

- WHEN will the transfer of the medical records take place?

- WHERE will the medical records be transferred to?

The answers to WHAT, HOW, and WHEN will depend on the transfer method selected. The answer to WHERE will depend on factors such as the transfer method, availability of storage areas, and type of storage. The perpetual transfer method is the most common transfer method. The *perpetual transfer method* involves continually removing medical records as they are no longer needed.

Medical records of patients not seen in a health facility for a certain period of time, such as one year, will be removed from the file area. A date for transfer is established, and personnel and equipment necessary for the transfer should be available. If the medical records are to be transferred to another facility or another location within the medical facility, adequate storage space and filing equipment should be available before the transfer takes place.

ACTIVE VERSUS INACTIVE MEDICAL RECORDS

Active medical records are those that are being used frequently in providing care to the patient. The availability of medical records in treating patients assures continuity of care and serves as a reference for the physician. Active records should be kept in a file storage area where they are easily accessible. *Inactive* medical records are records that are not frequently used. A patient may have moved, died, or stopped being seen by the physician or hospital.

The medical facility should have a policy for handling inactive records in order to accommodate the expanding files. For all practical purposes, the chief criterion for determining inactivity is the available space for efficient storage of newer medical records. In one medical facility, five years since last use may be the designated time for classifying medical records as inactive. Another medical facility may have a shortage of storage space, and may designate two years since last use as the standard. For example, an individual may have been a patient in the hospital but not needed hospitalization within the specified two-year time period. Therefore, the medical record has become inactive.

An orthopedic surgeon may have treated a patient for a fractured hip. Once the hip healed, the patient returned to the primary care physician and did not visit the orthopedic surgeon again. If the medical facility's plan states medical records will be inactive if a patient has not been seen for one year, the medical record at the orthopedist's office becomes inactive at that time.

Inactive medical records may be stored in another area of the facility, commercially stored, microfilmed, or stored on optical or magnetic disk. Location of these records should be noted in the master patient index in order to avoid unnecessary searching of files.

Student Name _____

Check Your Knowledge

Directions:
Complete the following sentences by writing the word(s) that best complete each sentence on the line provided.

1. Medical records that are used frequently for patient appointments are called

    _____.

2. The recommended number of years to retain medical records is

    _____.

3. Medical records of deceased patients are known as

    _____.

4. A procedure that ensures that all borrowed medical records are accounted for is known as

    _____.

5. A form for recording information about the record when it is borrowed is a(n)

    _____.

6. Four key words for questions to be answered before transfer of medical records are

    _____.

7. An OUT guide is a means of

    _____.

8. Checking on medical records not returned within a certain time frame is known as

    _____.

9. The maximum recommended time a medical record should be borrowed is

    _____.

10. A transfer method that specifies removing medical records continually as they are no longer needed is called

    _____.

11. In setting their retention policy when there is no state law governing the time for retention of medical records, medical facilities should consider the

    _____.

12. A number on the patient medical record folder which can be scanned to speed the chart tracking process is called

    _____.

Unit 7

Computer-Assisted Filing

Computer applications for medical facilities were first used by hospitals for financial and administrative purposes. Today computers are being used more and more in physician's offices and other medical facilities. Computers primarily store and distribute information. They allow data to be collected and then shared throughout the medical facility. For example, on the patient's first visit, pertinent data such as name, address, birth date, and insurance carrier are collected. This data could serve as the master patient index and also be shared with the billing office. Use of computers saves time and reduces errors because information will be entered into the computer only once. In addition, patients are not asked the same questions more than once.

Once a database is created, a variety of reports can be generated. A **database** is a collection of related information or files that may be used to create reports regarding a facility's activities. A **report** is a summary of information. Examples of reports would be a list of unpaid patient accounts or a summary of patient visits each day for a month. This information may be viewed on the screen or printed.

Three types of computer applications used in medical facilities include administrative, financial, and clinical applications.

ADMINISTRATIVE APPLICATIONS

A wide variety of administrative computer applications are available. Both hospitals and physician's offices will benefit from the use of administrative databases. Some of the administrative databases that will be discussed in *Medical Filing* are appointment scheduling, patient registration, and record location and tracking. In addition to these three areas, various departments within the hospital and clinic setting such as physical therapy, x-ray, and laboratory might also computerize their functions. Computerized inventory control of patient supplies and drugs provides an efficient method for ordering and keeping track of these materials.

Information sharing is a key to successful health care data systems. For example, on admission basic patient information will be collected. When a drug is ordered for the patient, the computer not only communicates with the pharmacy to fill the order but also debits the pharmacy inventory and creates an entry on the patient's bill. Later on, if someone wishes to do research on that particular drug, information concerning the patient would be available.

Appointment Scheduling

Appointments can be made, changed, cancelled and confirmed using a computer. In a physician's office or clinic, each physician has an individual appointment slot, and the computerized appointment book is searched for available openings. A daily list of appointments can be generated. This list will be used to retrieve medical records for appointments, to inform the physician of the day's schedule, and to allow personnel to call patients to remind them of their appointments.

Patient Registration

On the first visit, the medical facility requests patients to complete a form that asks for personal, insurance, and employer information. This information is then entered into the computer and can be added to or changed whenever necessary. When a numeric method for storing medical records is used, the computer can assign patient numbers. For example, if numbers are assigned consecutively and a patient comes to the medical facility for the first time, the computer would assign the next available number.

The patient registration database is shared with other departments such as the business office and medical records. The business office will add charges as necessary and then generate a patient bill. In medical records, the database may be used as a master patient index.

It is important that all information be accurate and correctly entered into the computer. Incorrect information is not of any value and may even be harmful to the patient. It is also time-consuming to correct wrong information. In a hospital, the patient registration database can produce admission forms, daily admission and discharge lists, and a variety of statistical data such as number of beds occupied, types of procedures performed, and most common diagnoses of patients.

Record Location and Tracking

A computerized record location and tracking system will provide information as to the location of a medical record at any given point. It can be used to check out records, to track overdue medical records, and to provide information about the past activity of a patient's medical record. A list of overdue medical records can be generated to make follow-up more efficient. An advantage of a computerized tracking system is that OUT guides would not be necessary. However, no tracking system will improve efficiency if all personnel do not consistently enter the information into the computer.

FINANCIAL APPLICATIONS

Financial applications are primarily related to billing and accounts management. There are many databases available, and a medical facility must determine their needs before selecting the appropriate database for their computer financial applications. Financial databases include billing, patient ledger, daily charges, and claims processing.

Billing

Patient's bills may be generated using the computerized accounting system. A bill can be generated to include all the necessary information for submission to the insurance company for reimbursement to the patient, physician, or hospital. This bill will be submitted along with an appropriate insurance form. An example of a computerized patient bill is shown in Figure 7.1.

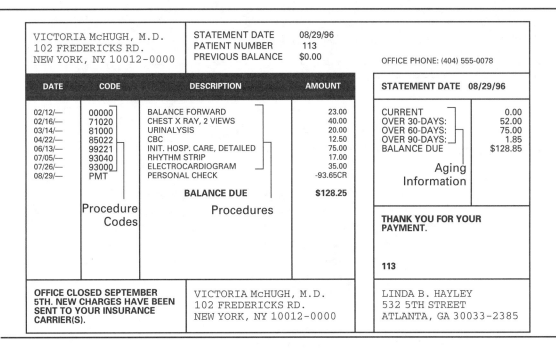

Figure 7.1 Computerized Patient Bill

Patient Ledger Cards

A patient ledger contains personal patient information such as address, insurance carriers, employer, and phone numbers, plus a listing of procedures and dates, charges, payments and adjustments. Computerized patient ledgers may contain additional information and can be customized to meet the health care facility's needs. Figure 7.2 shows a patient ledger card produced by a computer.

Figure 7.2
Computerized
Patient Ledger Card

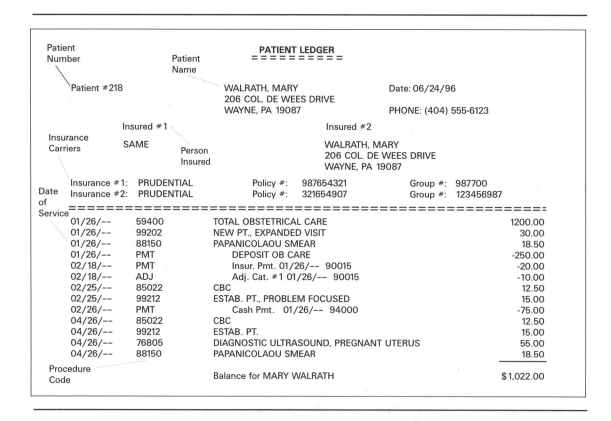

```
Patient
Number                            PATIENT LEDGER
                      Patient    = = = = = = = = = =
                      Name

      Patient #218               WALRATH, MARY              Date: 06/24/96
                                 206 COL. DE WEES DRIVE
                                 WAYNE, PA 19087            PHONE: (404) 555-6123

               Insured #1                        Insured #2
Insurance
Carriers       SAME                              WALRATH, MARY
                      Person                     206 COL. DE WEES DRIVE
                      Insured                    WAYNE, PA 19087

       Insurance #1:  PRUDENTIAL      Policy #:  987654321      Group #:  987700
Date   Insurance #2:  PRUDENTIAL      Policy #:  321654907      Group #:  123456987
of
Service ==============================================================
      01/26/--   59400    TOTAL OBSTETRICAL CARE                    1200.00
      01/26/--   99202    NEW PT., EXPANDED VISIT                     30.00
      01/26/--   88150    PAPANICOLAOU SMEAR                          18.50
      01/26/--   PMT      DEPOSIT OB CARE                           -250.00
      02/18/--   PMT      Insur. Pmt. 01/26/--  90015                -20.00
      02/18/--   ADJ      Adj. Cat. #1 01/26/--  90015               -10.00
      02/25/--   85022    CBC                                        12.50
      02/25/--   99212    ESTAB. PT., PROBLEM FOCUSED                15.00
      02/26/--   PMT      Cash Pmt.  01/26/--  94000                -75.00
      04/26/--   85022    CBC                                        12.50
      04/26/--   99212    ESTAB. PT.                                 15.00
      04/26/--   76805    DIAGNOSTIC ULTRASOUND, PREGNANT UTERUS     55.00
      04/26/--   88150    PAPANICOLAOU SMEAR                         18.50
Procedure                                                          _____
Code                     Balance for MARY WALRATH              $1,022.00
```

Daily Charges

On a daily basis, a medical facility may obtain a computerized report of all payments, charges, and adjustments. In addition, information may be available on the number of patients seen in a medical facility on any given day, their names, and procedures charged to each. This information may also be available on a weekly or monthly basis. Figure 7.3 shows a daily charge report.

Figure 7.3
Daily Charge Report

```
                    DAILY JOURNAL OF CHARGES AND PAYMENTS
                                  05/20/96

PAT  NAME                    DATE      PROCEDURE                         N-SVS    CHARGE        PAYMENT
NO

100  ALLAN, ROBERT          0502--    32000  THORACOCENTESIS               8    $  640.00    $    0.00
100                         0520--    36800  INTRAVASCULAR-CANNULIZATION   1    $  110.00    $   50.00
100                         0520--    71020  CHEST X RAY, 2 VIEWS          1    $   30.00    $    5.00
100                         0501--    83498  HYDROXYPOGESTERONE-17         4    $  120.00    $   10.00
100                         0520--    83020  HEMOGLOBIN                    1    $   20.00    $    0.00
100                         0520--    99301  NURSING HOME VISIT, STRAIGHT
100                                          FORWARD ASSESSMENT            1    $   20.00    $    0.00
100                                   999.2  ADJ 90450 830520 830520       0    $  -20.00    $    0.00
102  BROWN, NAOMI           0520--    999.2  ADJ 830520 830520 36800       0    $ -110.00    $  -50.00
102                         0504--    80019  MULTICHANNEL TEST-19          1    $   54.00    $   24.00
103  CARDEN, ANNETTE L      0520--    99396  ANNUAL CHECK UP               4    $  300.00    $   50.00
103                         0520--    999.2  ADJ 830504 830512 90080       0    $ -300.00    $  -50.00
103                         0520--    92950  CARDIOPULMONARY RESUSCITATION 1    $  100.00    $    0.00
                                      93510  FEMORAL CATHETER              1    $   50.00    $   25.00
                                      81000  URINALYSIS                    1    $    9.75    $    0.00

MODE         NUMBER          TOTAL

0   CASH          9      $     0.00
1   CHECK         1      $     5.00
2   MONEY ORDER   1      $    10.00
3   VISA          1      $     0.00
4   MASTERCARD    2      $    49.00
5   INSURANCE     0      $     0.00
6   ADJUSTMENT    0      $     0.00
                                              TOTALS

         CHARGES  $1023.75     PAYMENTS  $64     ADJUSTMENTS  $0.00     NO OF PATIENTS  3
```

Claims Processing

Transmitting claims in a timely manner is as important as keeping accurate information regarding the patient account. The more quickly a claim is submitted to the payer, the sooner the health facility will receive payment. Electronic medical claim submission (EMCS) is used by many medical facilities when submitting claims. EMCS is the process of transmitting claims by way of data communications such as a telephone modem. In addition to providing faster reimbursement, it eliminates paper.

CLINICAL APPLICATIONS

Clinical computer applications pertain to data used to diagnose and treat patients. A computerized medical record documents the health care provided by physicians, nurses, physical therapists, and others involved in health care. To date, a totally paperless medical record does not exist, but advances are continually being made, and one may be seen in the near future.

Information stored in a database can be used to develop research reports. For example, information regarding the treatment and response to treatment of patients with cancer will assist the physician in making recommendations for future treatment. Files can also be searched for names of patients who are due for an annual physical so that they can be notified.

Computer-assisted diagnostic and treatment regimens are becoming very popular. For example, the dosage of many drugs used in the treatment of burns is calculated based on the height and weight of the patient and the percentage of total body surface area that is burned. In many large burn units, this is calculated by computer. Using the patient database, the physician simply enters the name of the drug into the computer, which then calculates the dosage.

HOSPITAL VERSUS PHYSICIAN'S OFFICE COMPUTER APPLICATIONS

With increased computer literacy and availability of more cost-effective computer equipment and software, both hospitals and physician's offices are utilizing computer applications. Personal computers (PCs) and local area networks (LANs) are making an impact on physician's offices. Use of a PC in a LAN allows information to be entered and shared from a variety of locations within an office.

Financial applications in all medical facilities are basically the same. Whether in a hospital, clinic, or physician's office, timely billing and processing of claims is important to the health facility's cash flow. It is sound financial management to know the income and expenses of the health facility on a routine basis. While the procedures may be different, the computer applications are similar.

In administrative applications the physician's office or clinic will utilize appointment scheduling more often than the hospital. However, hospital outpatient services such as lab and x-ray may utilize appointment scheduling, as well as planned admissions. Many hospital admissions are emergencies and therefore not scheduled appointments. Because hospitals are larger and medical records may be checked out to a variety of departments, chart tracking is used more in hospitals than in physician's offices.

Research is performed more widely in the hospitals so this administrative application of database would be utilized more frequently in hospitals than other settings.

SECURITY AND CONFIDENTIALITY

Security and confidentiality of computerized information are as important as with the paper medical record. Data and information are to be accessed only by authorized personnel. To assure that only authorized personnel access information, mechanisms need to be in place. For example, a password not known to anyone else should be assigned to each person needing access to the computer information. Each time the individual uses the system, the password must be entered. The password does not show on the screen so that anyone looking on does not have access to the password. If an incorrect password is entered, access to the system will be denied. To maintain security, a medical facility may want to routinely change passwords of employees. The success of the password in maintaining security depends on its not being shared with unauthorized persons.

Student Name

Check Your Knowledge

Directions:
In each of the following situations, identify the computer application involved by writing financial, administrative, or clinical on the line provided.

1. Personal information about a patient.

   _____

2. Personal information along with charges and payments.

   _____

3. Dr. Mario Soto's office calling Anytown Hospital to schedule Mary Larson for a mammogram.

   _____

4. Computer information on the physical therapy progress of Josh Moreno.

   _____

5. Dr. Emil Maddern's request for a list of all patients diagnosed with cancer during the past year.

   _____

Directions:
In each of the following situations, identify the computer application involved AND, if appropriate, the database that would be utilized.

6. Anytown Medical Center received a request for copies of the medical record of Frances Cavetti from Anytown Hospital. The medical record was not in the storage area, and no OUT guide was in place.

   _____

7. Metropolitan Medical office has seven physicians. Maria Louvar phoned to arrange a time to see Dr. J. P. Lopez for a postsurgical check up.

   _____

8. Gynecologist Associates received information regarding intrauterine devices (IUDs) that indicated they were not as safe as once thought. They wish to inform patients who have had an IUD inserted.

   _____

This exercise continues on the following page.

9. Miami Clinic's medical records are computerized. The results of a chest x-ray are necessary for further treatment of Charles Lang.

_____

10. Anytown Medical Center requests a breakdown of daily charges for the last week of September.

_____

Answers

CHECK YOUR UNDERSTANDING ANSWERS

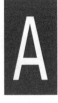

Rule 1 (p. 17)

		Key Unit	Unit 2	Unit 3
1	1.	MEIER	JOHN	
4	2.	MEIR	JOHN	ROBERT
6	3.	MEIRS	J	ROBERT
3	4.	MEIR	J	R
5	5.	MEIR	JULIA	
7	6.	MIERS	JULIA	A
2	7.	MEIERS	JOAN	K

Rules 2, 3, and 4 (p. 19)

		Key Unit	Unit 2	Unit 3
6	1.	LYNCHWEBER	MAGDALENA	
2	2.	DCENZO	CARLOS	
4	3.	LIU	ICHEN	
3	4.	DEANDRE	JOS	THOMAS
7	5.	STVINCENT	WILL	M
1	6.	DAMICO	JOE	THOS
5	7.	LLOYD	M	CARMEN

Rule 5 (p. 20)

		Key Unit	Unit 2	Unit 3	Unit 4
5	1.	PEREZ	VICTOR	S	DR
1	2.	GOEDKEN	TOM	K	FATHER
6	3.	SISTER	LORETTA		
3	4.	HERNANDEZ	JOSE	F	SENIOR
2	5.	HERNANDEZ	JOSE	F	II
7	6.	TIRADO	CLARK	PhD	PROF
4	7.	KING	HARALD	V	

Rule 6 (p. 21)

3	1.	Ms. Amanda K. Fransen, 1120 E. Main, Lansing, IA
7	2.	Paul John Lansing, St. Paul, MN
2	3.	Amanda K. Fransen, 112 W. Main, Lansing, IA
4	4.	Paul John Lansing, St. Paul, MI
1	5.	Miss Anna Maria Franks
5	6.	Mr. D.M. LaBrie, Ely, NV
6	7.	Delora LaBrie, 19 Pine Tree Ave., Ely, MN

Phonetic Filing (p. 23)

	Name	Phonetic Code
1.	Chase, Vivian	C000
2.	DeGrotte, Alma	D263
3.	Gjerdahl, Felicia R.	G634
4.	Kollar, Rosa	K460
5.	Schrader, Laurie	S636
6.	Toutloff, Andrew	T341
7.	Whittington, Lee	W352

Unit 3   **CHECK YOUR UNDERSTANDING ANSWERS**

Assigning a Patient Number (p. 31)

2	1.	Prepare a patient card
1	2.	Enter patient name in accession book
3	3.	Write patient number on medical record

Retrieving a Medical Record (p. 31)

3	1.	Retrieve medical record from file
2	2.	Locate patient number on patient card
1	3.	Locate patient card in alphabetic card file

Consecutive Numeric Filing   (p. 33)

1. 330172
2. 330712
3. 337012
4. 337021
5. 457813
6. 458731
7. 459313

Terminal-Digit Filing   (p. 34)

1.	36-34-18	5.	35-34-81
2.	23-43-18	6.	12-35-81
3.	23-44-18	7.	13-35-81
4.	24-44-18	8.	23-43-81

Middle-Digit Filing (p. 35)

1.	23-89-56	5.	23-92-51
2.	32-89-56	6.	23-92-56
3.	32-89-57	7.	32-92-56
4.	23-92-50	8.	24-93-56

Unit 4 **CHECK YOUR UNDERSTANDING ANSWERS**

Alphabetic Cross-Referencing (p. 43)

1. LACY ANNA MARIA   LACY BILL MRS
    SEE: LACY ANNA MARIA

2. TIEN SHENG   SHENG TIEN
    SEE: TIEN SHENG

3. HANSEN IOLA   HANSON IOLA
    SEE: HANSEN IOLA

4. NICHOLASHANS CARRIE   HANS CARRIE NICHOLAS
    SEE: NICHOLASHANS CARRIE

5. THOMAS GEORGE   GEORGE THOMAS
    SEE: THOMAS GEORGE

Unit 5 **CHECK YOUR UNDERSTANDING ANSWERS**

Alphabetic Color Coding (p. 50)

	Position 3	Position 4
1.	white	blue
2.	green	brown
3.	light blue	grey
4.	green	brown
5.	yellow	blue

Numeric Color Coding (p. 52)

	Primary	Secondary	Tertiary
1.	pink-blue	light blue-red	pink-white
2.	pink-blue	light blue-light blue	pink-white
3.	pink-red	red-light blue	pink-white
4.	pink-light blue	white-white	pink-blue
5.	light blue-pink	white-pink	pink-red

Unit 6   **CHECK YOUR UNDERSTANDING ANSWERS**

Charge-Out Procedures   (p. 61)

1.   follow-up
2.   requisition form
3.   OUT guide
4.   false
5.   tickler file
6.   false
7.   a. improves record access

   b. faciliates record retrieval

   c. reduces incidence of misplaced records

Glossary

G

accession ledger a record of the consecutive numbers assigned to patients.

alphabetic filing records are arranged according to the letters of the alphabet.

automated tracking system computerized system identifying the location of medical records at any given point of time.

bar code represents numbers which can be scanned into a computer.

color-coded filing system a color is assigned to each letter (in alphabetic filing) or number (in numeric filing).

computerized patient record records are stored on a computer to enhance and facilitate communication among health care providers at various locations and distance.

consecutive numeric filing system arrangement of medical records by assigned numbers, starting the lowest number and ending with the highest. Also known as straight numeric.

cross-referencing an aid that indicates another way a medical record may be filed.

database collection of related information or files that may be used to create reports.

file guides dividers that guide the way to the location of the record being retrieved.

follow-up checking on the return of borrowed medical records within a reasonable length of time.

indexing selecting the file segment under which a record will be billed.

master patient index a card file or computerized file that contains information on all patients treated by a health facility.

medical record permanent written document containing pertinent facts about a patient's illnesses and treatments.

microfilming photographic process that reduces a document to a very small size.

middle-digit filing numbers are grouped according to pairs of digits with the primary numbers being the middle two digits.

numeric filing a number is assigned to each record and filed according to one of the various numeric sequences.

optical disk storage uses a laser to etch data onto a permanent surface such as prepared glass and can store vast amount of paper information on a single disk.

out-guides a card, folder, or sheet of paper temporarily inserted in the file to replace a medical record that has been removed.

phonetic filing a filing system by which all surnames that sound alike but are spelled differently are filed together by using a code number which represents key letters.

records control procedures used to keep track of medical records.

report summary of information

requisition a request for a medical record usually using a specific requisition form.

serial numbering patient receives a new number at the time of each visit.

serial-unit numbering patient receives a new number at the time of each visit but the previous medical record is brought forward and incorporated into the record with the new number.

statute of Limitations a specific time frame for bringing legal action.

tab a portion of the folder that extends beyond the regular height or width of the folder.

terminal-digit groups numbers into units containing two digits each. The digits are read from right to left.

tickler file serves a reminder that specific action is to taken on a specific date.

unit numbering patient is assigned a patient number on the first visit and retains the same number for subsequent visits.

Index

NOTES:

NOTES:

NOTES:

NOTES:

NOTES:

Cards

C

Sonny L. D' Hanes

1024 Norway Drive

Ely, MN 55731

ALPHABETIC

Emi T. Di Cello

102 Beacon Hill Drive

Fargo, ND 58102

ALPHABETIC

Steven L. Mac Clure

19041 Dows Rd. NE

Cedar Rapids, IA 52402

ALPHABETIC

Tomas K. de Rosette

Box 452

Fairfax, IA 52228

ALPHABETIC

Norma Rae Garcia-Reiter

Rt. 1

Fairmont, MN 56031

ALPHABETIC

Dr. Mariann Reiter

14000 Club Road

Whitefish Bay, WI 53217

ALPHABETIC

John P. St. Claire

1581 Sparrow Rd.

St. Louis, MO 63115

ALPHABETIC

Sally K. Fried-Marr

3891 Hillcrest Drive

Kansas City, MO 64131

ALPHABETIC

Sam C. D'Elia

750 N. 150th Street

Aberdeen, SD 57401

ALPHABETIC

Virginia Hair-De Narr

357 Lakewood Drive

Madison, TN 37115

ALPHABETIC

Lidia K. Mc Bride

125 Bluebird Road

Appleton, WI 54914

ALPHABETIC

Carlos L. Reiter, Sr.

2000 Cains Hill Drive

St. Louis, MO 63367

ALPHABETIC

Osami M. Friedman

501 Maple Street

Topeka, KS 66614

ALPHABETIC

Irene N. Feng

199 Marigold Avenue

Phoenix, AZ 85016

ALPHABETIC

Rev. Robin K. Scott

29 Montery Drive

Madison, TN 37115

ALPHABETIC

Lydia A. Reiter-Lloyd

1259 David Court

Miami, FL 34002

ALPHABETIC

Mr. Carlos L. Reiter, II

1044 4th Ave. So.

Manden, ND 58554

ALPHABETIC

Prof. Darryl Reiter

894 Henderson Avenue

Fremont, MI 49412

ALPHABETIC

Dr. Clara E. Rodriquez

8182 Heather Lane

Elgin, IL 60123

ALPHABETIC

Monica Rae de la Mater

4813 Belmont Avenue

Lansing, IL 60438

ALPHABETIC

Sister Matilde

829 W. Highland

Indianapolis, IN 46250

ALPHABETIC

Ms. Sandra Ann De Narr

2481 Sunshine Road

Madison, WI 523707

ALPHABETIC

Mayor Perry F. Valdez

14621 Lincolnshire Drive

Omaha, NE 68144

ALPHABETIC

Kevin Jay Van Houten

1432 1st Street

Little Rock, AR 72211

ALPHABETIC

Mr. Tomas V. Saint James

245 South Ridge Drive

San Antonio, TX 78240

ALPHABETIC

Mrs. Mary-Lou K. Reiter

R.R. 2

Ely, IA 52227

ALPHABETIC

Father Victor R. Phillips

1141 Spanish Road

Torrance, CA 90501

ALPHABETIC

| TERMINAL-/MIDDLE-DIGIT | 05-00-75 |
| CONSECUTIVE NUMBER | 50075 |

Father Victor R. Phillips

1141 Spanish Road

Torrance, CA 90501

NUMERIC

Sister Catherine Jensen

5001 Adam St. So.

Minneapolis, MN 55410

ALPHABETIC

Queen Margaret

100 Main Street

Belleville, IL 62220

ALPHABETIC

Celia R. Mac Millan

305 Walker Avenue

Battle Creek, MI 49015

ALPHABETIC

| TERMINAL-/MIDDLE-DIGIT | 00-89-16 |
| CONSECUTIVE NUMBER | 8916 |

Celia R. Mac Millan

305 Walker Avenue

Battle Creek, MI 49015

NUMERIC

Terminal-/Middle-Digit	00-87-16	Terminal-/Middle-digit	27-13-75
Consecutive Number	8716	Consecutive Number	271375

Sonny L. D' Hanes

1024 Norway Drive

Ely, MN 55731

NUMERIC

Emi T. Di Cello

102 Beacon Hill Drive

Fargo, ND 58102

NUMERIC

Terminal-/Middle-Digit	78-05-28	Terminal-/Middle-Digit	87-05-28
Consecutive Number	780528	Consecutive Number	870528

Steven L. Mac Clure

19041 Dows Rd. NE

Cedar Rapids, IA 52402

NUMERIC

Tomas K. de Rosette

Box 452

Fairfax, IA 52228

NUMERIC

Terminal-/Middle-Digit	29-13-75	Terminal-/Middle-Digit	35-05-28
Consecutive Number	291375	Consecutive Number	350528

Norma Rae Garcia-Reiter

Rt. 1

Fairmont, MN 56031

NUMERIC

Dr. Mariann Reiter

14000 Club Road

Whitefish Bay, WI 53217

NUMERIC

Terminal-/Middle-Digit	01-90-15	Terminal-/Middle-Digit	25-13-75
Consecutive Number	19015	Consecutive Number	251375

John P. St. Claire

1581 Sparrow Rd.

St. Louis, MO 63115

NUMERIC

Sally K. Fried-Marr

3891 Hillcrest Drive

Kansas City, MO 64131

NUMERIC

Terminal-/Middle-Digit 65-25-75	Terminal-/Middle-Digit 68-02-29
Consecutive Number 652575	Consecutive Number 680229
Sam C. D'Elia	Virginia Hair-De Narr
750 N. 150th Street	357 Lakewood Drive
Aberdeen, SD 57401	Madison, TN 37115
NUMERIC	NUMERIC

Terminal-/Middle-Digit 65-05-28	Terminal-/Middle-Digit 67-01-29
Consecutive Number 650528	Consecutive Number 670129
Lidia K. Mc Bride	Carlos L. Reiter, Sr.
125 Bluebird Road	2000 Cains Hill Drive
Appleton, WI 54914	St. Louis, MO 63367
NUMERIC	NUMERIC

Terminal-/Middle-Digit 66-01-29	Terminal-/Middle-Digit 65-01-29
Consecutive Number 660129	Consecutive Number 650129
Osami M. Friedman	Irene N. Feng
501 Maple Street	199 Marigold Avenue
Topeka, KS 66614	Phoenix, AZ 85016
NUMERIC	NUMERIC

Terminal-/Middle-Digit 98-45-75	Terminal-/Middle-Digit 22-05-28
Consecutive Number 984575	Consecutive Number 220528
Rev. Robin K. Scott	Lydia A. Reiter-Lloyd
29 Montery Drive	1259 David Court
Madison, TN 37115	Miami, FL 34002
NUMERIC	NUMERIC

TERMINAL-/MIDDLE-DIGIT 45-05-28	TERMINAL-/MIDDLE-DIGIT 03-90-15
CONSECUTIVE NUMBER 450528	CONSECUTIVE NUMBER 39015

Mr. Carlos L. Reiter, II

1044 4th Ave. So.

Manden, ND 58554

NUMERIC

Sister Matilde

829 W. Highland

Indianapolis, IN 46250

NUMERIC

TERMINAL-/MIDDLE-DIGIT 02-90-15	TERMINAL-/MIDDLE-DIGIT 00-89-15
CONSECUTIVE NUMBER 29015	CONSECUTIVE NUMBER 8915

Prof. Darryl Reiter

894 Henderson Avenue

Fremont, MI 49412

NUMERIC

Ms. Sandra Ann De Narr

2481 Sunshine Road

Madison, WI 52370

NUMERIC

TERMINAL-/MIDDLE-DIGIT 32-90-15	TERMINAL-/MIDDLE-DIGIT 33-45-75
CONSECUTIVE NUMBER 329015	CONSECUTIVE NUMBER 334575

Dr. Clara E. Rodriquez

8182 Heather Lane

Elgin, IL 60123

NUMERIC

Mayor Perry F. Valdez

14621 Lincolnshire Drive

Omaha, NE 68144

NUMERIC

TERMINAL-/MIDDLE-DIGIT 37-45-75	TERMINAL-/MIDDLE-DIGIT 00-80-15
CONSECUTIVE NUMBER 374575	CONSECUTIVE NUMBER 8015

Monica Rae de la Mater

4813 Belmont Avenue

Lansing, IL 60438

NUMERIC

Kevin Jay Van Houten

1432 1st Street

Little Rock, AR 72211

NUMERIC

Terminal-/Middle-Digit   21-00-15

Consecutive Number   210015

Mr. Tomas V. Saint James

245 South Ridge Drive

San Antonio, TX 78240

NUMERIC

Terminal-/Middle-Digit   97-45-75

Consecutive Number   974575

Sister Catherine Jensen

5001 Adam St. So.

Minneapolis, MN 55410

NUMERIC

Terminal-/Middle-Digit   10-90-15

Consecutive Number   109015

Mrs. Mary-Lou K. Reiter

R.R. 2

Ely, IA 52227

NUMERIC

Terminal-/Middle-Digit   23-90-15

Consecutive Number   239015

Queen Margaret

100 Main Street

Belleville, IL 62220

NUMERIC

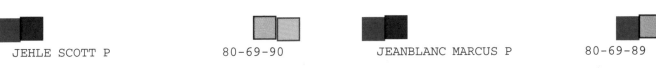

JEHLE SCOTT P   80-69-90

JEANBLANC MARCUS P   80-69-89

COLOR CODING

COLOR CODING

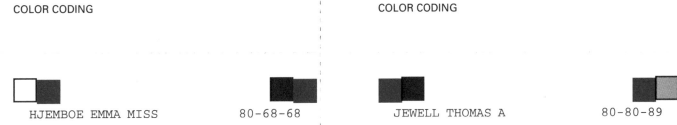

HJEMBOE EMMA MISS   80-68-68

JEWELL THOMAS A   80-80-89

COLOR CODING

COLOR CODING

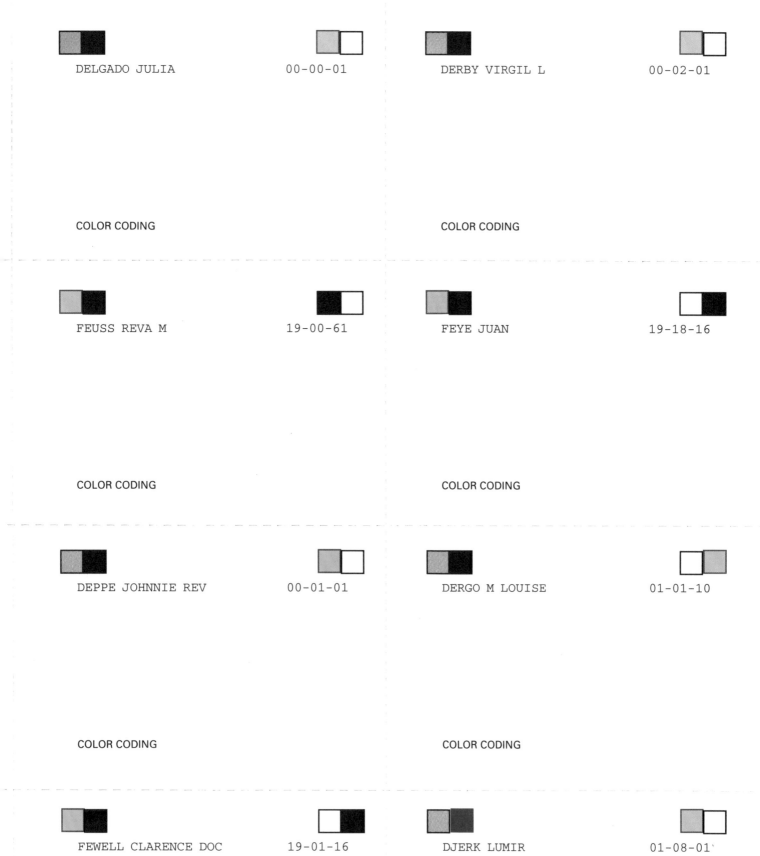

DELGADO JULIA   00-00-01

COLOR CODING

DERBY VIRGIL L   00-02-01

COLOR CODING

FEUSS REVA M   19-00-61

COLOR CODING

FEYE JUAN   19-18-16

COLOR CODING

DEPPE JOHNNIE REV   00-01-01

COLOR CODING

DERGO M LOUISE   01-01-10

COLOR CODING

FEWELL CLARENCE DOC   19-01-16

COLOR CODING

DJERK LUMIR   01-08-01

COLOR CODING

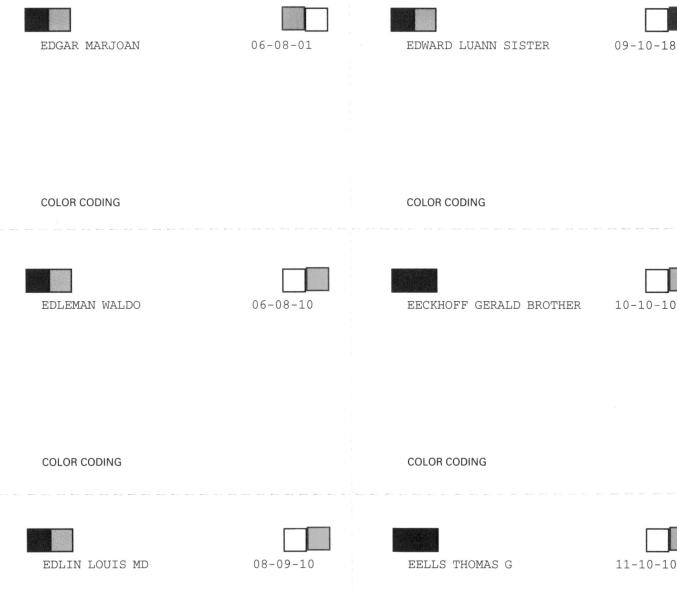

EDGAR MARJOAN   06-08-01

COLOR CODING

EDWARD LUANN SISTER   09-10-18

COLOR CODING

EDLEMAN WALDO   06-08-10

COLOR CODING

EECKHOFF GERALD BROTHER   10-10-10

COLOR CODING

EDLIN LOUIS MD   08-09-10

COLOR CODING

EELLS THOMAS G   11-10-10

COLOR CODING

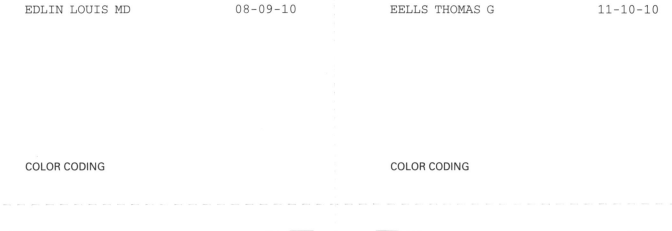

EDMOND KIM MS   09-09-10

COLOR CODING

FENG LIN   11-11-16

COLOR CODING

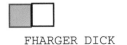 FHARGER DICK

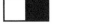 19-06-68

 HEARN ANGELIQUE

 20-06-68

COLOR CODING

COLOR CODING

 FERNANDEZ HAZEL MS

 11-16-16

 HEATH YOKO S

 19-08-68

COLOR CODING

COLOR CODING

 FETZER CARLOS

 16-18-16

 HEATHMAN OLIVIA

 61-16-86

COLOR CODING

COLOR CODING

 HEBEL BENJI JUDGE

 61-18-68

 HECK CHINGYU

 68-68-68

COLOR CODING

COLOR CODING

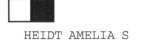 HEIDT AMELIA S   69-68-86   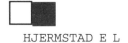 HJERMSTAD E L   80-68-89

COLOR CODING

COLOR CODING

MACKENZIE STEPHEN J II   10-00-46   MACKENZIE STEPHANIE O   00-01-64

25   FINAL PROJECT   **28**   FINAL PROJECT

BELDINGSCHMITT BETH   10-10-00   MILOWSKI BRYANT W MR   46-01-46

26   FINAL PROJECT   **29**   FINAL PROJECT

MACKEY MARY JUDE SISTER   64-01-46   MCKENZIE SUSAN PROF   69-25-98

27   FINAL PROJECT   **30**   FINAL PROJECT

Christopher P. O'Brien, Sr.   46-01-00

4531 West 22nd Street

Valley, FL 32244

1   FINAL PROJECT

Brother Donovan   98-23-98

8021 Notre Dame

Valley, FL 32244

2   FINAL PROJECT

Vincent R. Gutierrez   01-46-64

630 Prairie Drive Northeast

North Valley, FL 32250

3   FINAL PROJECT

Mario L. Bryant, Ph.D.   98-24-98

421 First Street South

Valley, FL 32244

4   FINAL PROJECT

Mr. Yoko Belding   46-10-00

24128 Hickory Lane

Palm Harbor, FL 34682

5   FINAL PROJECT

Lu-Yin Lan   00-00-46

325 Dover Lane

North VaLLey, FL 32244

6   FINAL PROJECT

Stephen J. Mackenzie, II   10-00-46

1000 Lakeshore Drive

Cocoa, FL 32922

7   FINAL PROJECT

Beth Belding-Schmitt   10-10-00

2250 Park Lane

Palm Harbor, FL 34582

8   FINAL PROJECT

DONOVAN BROTHER   98-23-98   LAN LUYIN   00-00-46

17   FINAL PROJECT   **21**   FINAL PROJECT

GUTIERREZ VINCENT R   01-46-64   YULAN CHRIS LU   89-25-98

18   FINAL PROJECT   **22**   FINAL PROJECT

BRYANT MARIO L PHD   98-24-98   HOPE ADRIANNE KAY   01-00-64

19   FINAL PROJECT   **23**   FINAL PROJECT

BELDING YOKO MR   46-10-00   MACLACHLAN IRENE J MD   64-01-00

20   FINAL PROJECT   **24**   FINAL PROJECT

FINAL PROJECT

FINAL PROJECT

FINAL PROJECT

FINAL PROJECT

FINAL PROJECT

FINAL PROJECT

FINAL PROJECT

FINAL PROJECT